" 'Kill me, kill me, kill me! I don't want to live, and I can't do it myself! Oh, please, kill me, Mother!' "

"There on his knees before me, his arms encircling my legs, our 12-year-old son and only child begged me to take his life. . . ."

Billy is the only son of Bill and Jessie Foy. He is now a healthy teenager. But from birth to his 14th year, he was the victim of childhood schizophrenia.

Gone Is Shadows' Child is a powerful testimony of a mother's love and courage—and the story of the little-known biochemical treatment that restored Billy Foy to sanity.

It presents a clear ray of hope in what has long been a dark wasteland of human suffering and medical ignorance.

GONE IS
SHADOWS' CHILD

Jessie Gray Foy

▲
PYRAMID BOOKS • NEW YORK

GONE IS SHADOWS' CHILD

A PYRAMID BOOK
Published by arrangement with Logos International

Pyramid edition published September, 1971
    Second printing February, 1972

Library of Congress Catalog Card Number: 72-111085

Printed in the United States of America

SBN 912106-08-5

PYRAMID BOOKS are published by Pyramid Communications, Inc. Its trademarks consisting of the word "Pyramid" and the portrayal of a pyramid, are registered in the United States Patent Office.

Pyramid Communications, Inc., 919 Third Avenue, New York, New York 10022, U.S.A.

I dedicate this story to my son, whose courage is boundless. To my husband, whose patience and strength of character helped me unceasingly.

To the memory of my father, a man whose unselfishness was an example of true love.

Shadows

Deep shadows crossed our young son's life,
Denied him peace, confused his mind.
What caused the threatening shadows?
What answers could we find?

They wished to claim our treasure,
But we could not let this be;
As long as love and life were ours,
We fought to set him free.

We looked, we searched for answers,
Groping, stumbling, day by day,
Until we found the right ones
To ease his troubled way.

Now we are rejoicing,
His spirit grows, breaks free.
As shadows are receding,
The change is there to see.

Beyond the veil of darkness
There dwelt a wholesome child,
And when the shadows parted,
He came forth sweet and mild.

For all of you who suffer,
Who would an answer find,
Call up your strength and courage,
Come, seek true peace of mind.

You must be unrelenting,
Or they will crush you sure.
Take heart, now, hope is offered;
With patience you'll endure.

Observe the ways of shadows,
Evasive, fleeting, real.
Shake loose their cloaking darkness
And light will come to heal.

JESSIE GRAY FOY

Contents

Introduction

For many, perhaps most of its readers, this book may be the first they have read about schizophrenia written by an immediate family member of the sick person.

There are a number of these histories, two recent and somewhat similar ones being *This Stranger My Son* and *And Always Tomorrow*. During the last century, at least one hundred books have been written in English by the victims of schizophrenia and other psychiatric illnesses. One of these accounts is Clifford Beers' famous *A Mind That Found Itself,* which resulted in the formation of the National Association of Mental Health; another is High Judge Daniel Schreber's *Memoirs of My Nervous Illness,* which was used by Freud as the basis for the psychoanalytic theory of paranoia.

The late Professor Carney Landis of Columbia has given the best survey of these books in his *Varieties of Psychopathological Experience.* Slightly earlier, Robert Sommer and I wrote "Autobiographies of Former Mental Patients," a paper emphasizing the great importance of these books and noting how few attempts had been made to study them systematically.

Since much has already been written about schizophrenia, one might ask whether there is need for any more. I believe that there is. *Gone Is Shadows' Child* fills that need, first, because it is a contemporary account of the effects of illness today; second, because I hope it will come to the attention of professionals involved in psychiatry; and third, because this particular story of a mother's struggle for her son's health has a more cheerful outcome than the two similar books already mentioned.

I shall not elaborate upon the author's account of how Billy began and sustained his improvement after years of illness. It is, of course, encouraging to find that Billy is now doing well; yet there is much else for all readers to ponder, especially those who are professionals in this field.

In the last two decades it has become almost commonplace, especially in North America, for some psychiatrists and others involved in treating schizophrenics to denounce the parents of children suffering from this illness. Such is the violence of some of these denunciations that even if they were founded upon substantial evidence, they would be considered slanderous in any except a medical setting. Parents have been accused of attempting to drive their children mad. Mothers have been the victims of a long, sustained, character assassination which has few parallels in medicine.

It seems likely that most psychiatrists don't believe these harsh accusations; yet, nevertheless, those who make them are allowed to continue doing so with remarkable complaisancy from their professional peers. It seems at least possible that clinicians and scientists have not been unduly distressed that some of the responsibility for the slow progress in exploring this illness should be dumped on the families of the ill, thus drawing attention from the shortcomings of psychiatry and its attendant sciences.

This cruel professional gossip has become so much a

part of the conventional wisdom that those who raise objections are frequently thought to be heretics, questioning the very foundations of psychiatry. Freud's sacred name has been invoked to support these accusatorial views, even though he probably would have repudiated them with alacrity. For much of Freud's life he was of the opinion that schizophrenia had a biochemical basis.

There is little evidence that the parents of children suffering from schizophrenia are either much better or worse than other parents; there is, however, a good deal of evidence that an ill child is likely to change the whole delicate fabric of family relationships, usually for the worse. Psychiatrists and psychologists have become the prisoners of their own strangely acquired theory, for the anxious, and often quite amiable, people who are the parents of the young schizophrenic do not appear to be as monstrous as the theory demands; and so there is a tendency to postpone or even evade diagnosis. The effect of failing to give any diagnosis, or of attaching such dubious labels as "a problem," or the highly ambiguous "emotional illness," is frequently even worse. The attempt to spare pain results in greater suffering for everyone.

The stresses of living with so hypersensitive a creature as Billy Foy must have been enormous. Young professionals who have not had children of their own ought to ponder the chapters dealing with the effect of Billy's illness on his parents. His early years were appalling for him and a nightmare for his parents. I can still recall the dismay suffered by my wife and myself when one night our little daughter had a nightmare. Her screams lasted for hours, so it seemed, even though the clock said it was only fifteen minutes. For the Foys there were whole nights of screaming.

Mrs. Foy has a number of keen observations and some pathetic illustrations of an aspect of schizophrenia which is often neglected in adults and seldom mentioned at all in children—the social relationships which go awry in this illness. From his earliest days Billy had great difficulty with his peers, much of it arising from his perceptual difficulties. Since it was hard for him to relate to those of his own age, he easily became a butt of humor, was bullied, and sometimes even brutally persecuted. He could not cope with more than a few people, even at home. He showed an almost total disregard for other people's feelings. This failure to form peer relationships receives little attention; yet it is probably a valuable clue to the nature and the progress of the illness. Maintaining such relationships depends on an accurate response to a great variety of cues, some of them very subtle. In schizophrenia, as its victims have repeatedly explained, these complex social cues become very difficult to cope with; yet as they begin to improve, these once insuperable barriers lessen, and, with recovery, gradually disappear.

Billy's story, tragic and horrifying in parts, is nevertheless an encouraging one. There are thousand of Billys all over the country whose parents are struggling desperately with this great illness. Like the Foys, many of them are also the victims of unproven psychiatric notions which have become part of the conventional wisdom. I hope this book will help to dispel these poorly founded ideas and encourage parents to urge their professional advisors to seek out more fruitful pathways, remembering what Florence Nightingale once called the first principle of a hospital—"to do the sick no harm."

As individuals, parents are unlikely to have much influence, but as members of an association such as the

American Schizophrenia Foundation they can and should make their voices heard loud and clear.

Humphry Osmond, MRCP, DPM
Director
Bureau of Research in Neurology and Psychiatry
State of New Jersey
Box 1000
Princeton, New Jersey 08540

November 17, 1969

Foreword

"Kill me, kill me, kill me! For God's sake, kill me! I don't want to live, and I can't do it myself! I am useless, hopeless! Oh, please, please, kill me, Mother!"

There on his knees before me, his arms encircling my legs, our twelve-year-old son and only child begged me to take his life. The tears were streaming down his contorted face as he implored me to relieve him from the emotional torment he had endured since his birth. In this pitiful cry his pain-racked spirit shouted for solace and relief. Truly he did not wish to die, but he could no longer endure his suffering.

I will never forget the look of stark terror in his eyes as he repeatedly screamed those hideous words at me. I turned my face away, for I could not bear to watch him. His outburst impaled my soul with anguish, and his cry of agony was beyond human belief. I bit into my lips to hold back my tears, and I felt myself trembling as I raised him from the floor, drawing his sobbing being close. I embraced him, and silently began to pray for the right words to comfort him.

I told him God wanted us to live; we could not kill ourselves or others. He had given us life, the most precious gift of all, for a purpose, not to be wasted. I told him we understood all that he was suffering; and we knew his feeling; and no matter how bad things were, we would not desert him. I pleaded with him to keep on trying, to have patience with himself and us.

I explained to my son how very proud we were of him and of the courage he had shown all these years. I said to him over and over that he must not give up, for we would not—ever; but my mind was deeply troubled. I promised, as I had countless times before, that everything would be all right. Somehow, through his excruciating torment, his disturbed and confused state of mind, he listened to me, and eventually composed himself.

What poor consolation words were to him! But words and love were all we had to offer our schizophrenic child then. As I held him close to me, I thought of other words, those of the twenty-third Psalm: "Yea, though I walk through the valley of the shadow of death, I will fear no evil; for Thou art with me." How often my mind had turned to these words for inspiration and confidence with each passing year as we labored to find an answer that would help our very ill child. For twelve years we had been grappling with the awesome shadows that threatened to destroy his life. *Shadows' child,* I thought, *held by the darkness of a disturbed spirit, living behind a veil, imprisoned in a tangle of unseen distortion.*

A thousand times we became disheartened and discouraged, confronted with our problem day after day. There were moments of great doubt for us and others, when we felt ourselves collapsing under the terrible strain of dealing with our son's emotional disabilities; but we kept searching persistently for help for him. My husband and I learned to sustain each other while keeping our worst thoughts hidden. If one of us lost his will to go on, the other gained determination; and in this way we maneuvered one another, as well as our son, through our ordeal. Each day we gave up. Each day we were more determined than ever to succeed. We lived on an unbalanced emotional see-saw, three people caught in the whirlwind preceding the hurricane's eye.

This is our story, every word the truth. It may seem incredible to some that our quest began fifteen years ago, and only now, thanks to man and God, a boy's life finally begins.

1

Before the Beginning and After the Beginning

"For goodness' sake, Bill, slow down! I know I'm sick, but you'll kill both of us before we get there, at this rate." My words were ignored as my husband raced me to the hospital.

"It's going to be all right, Jessie. Just hang on, you'll be fine," he said. I wondered if he was trying to convince me or himself. We had just left my doctor's office. The doctor was so shocked by my sudden violent illness that he left his other patients and followed us in his car.

It did not take long for him to find the cause of my frightful condition. I had diabetes mellitus, with severe diabetic acidosis, a dangerous state of affairs considering I was also four and a half months pregnant. As sick as I was, I cannot say I gave much thought to myself. The gravity of the situation hit me only when I heard the doctor and my husband conferring outside the door to my room, where I lay with needles in my arms and bottles hanging about.

"It's too soon to tell, Bill." The doctor's voice was guarded. "She is either going to get better or die, and right now I am not really sure which way things will go. The next few hours will tell the tale."

Die indeed, I thought. I absolutely refused and dismissed that possibility from my mind. But I could not so easily dismiss the possibility of losing our first child.

My husband and I had been married six years, and we were looking forward to our gift of love and joy. Were we to be robbed of it? I prayed not. My prayers were answered, and my unborn baby and I hung on to life as we conquered the first of many crises.

It was a couple of weeks before I was allowed to go home, and by that time I was taking my own insulin and feeling very well. During my stay in the hospital, my doctor insisted on a consultation with a specialist to determine what effect this previously undetected diabetic condition might have on my unborn child. After a brief examination, the specialist told me not to worry, that both of us would be fine. He was cheerful and confident, but a small nagging uneasiness—call it a premonition—kept tugging at my mind. I kept my fears to myself and determined to stay well for the baby's sake, as well as my own.

For a month or so, all remained quiet. I was just getting used to the diabetes when we discovered I had a kidney stone, too. This time, nature was on my side, and we disposed of the stone easily. The remainder of my wait passed without further complications, and eventually the hour of the great event arrived.

After the struggle of birth was over, I felt someone touching my shoulder, and I grunted, but did not open my eyes. I was too tired. I heard the voice of my husband reaching me through a sleepy haze.

"Jessie, Jessie, we had a boy!" There was the pride of fatherhood in his voice. I think I said something stupid, like "that's nice," and slipped back into a peaceful emptiness.

My son's introduction to this world had come at three minutes past 2 a.m. on February 20, 1954. The ravages of birth were evident as I first looked upon him. He arrived bruised and battered, with a large hematoma on the top of his head. The doctor told me much later that he had been hard to awaken, and, as he put it, had nearly drowned. To sustain his fragile grip on life, he was kept in an incubator his first three days.

I was unaware of my son's poor condition at first, and several times the following day I asked to see him. Everyone kept telling me he would be brought to my room soon. When he finally arrived, I lifted him up with mixed feelings of thankfulness and bewilderment that he was really ours. Suddenly I was aghast to see his reddish complexion turn a deep, purplish-blue color. I rang for the nurse, and she snatched him up in her arms, returning him to the nursery without a word of explanation. The next day they brought him back, and this time he did not change color, but he seemed to be strangling as he sucked his bottle.

When my doctor appeared, I asked him about Billy's color and his apparent feeding problems. He ignored my first question, but told me the child's tongue was held down by an extra piece of skin, and this would be clipped when he was circumcised in a few days. He also told me they were feeding him every two hours, instead of every four, alternating formula with sugar and water. When they tested his blood for evidence of diabetes, he proved not to have it.

Eventually Billy's color remained normal, and he took nourishment readily. When he really perked up, we were released from the hospital. Except for a slight nagging uneasiness I called "new motheritis," my concern for my baby relaxed. I felt the worst was over, but this thought was only temporary.

This tiny package of humanity, our little son, was a restless baby in the extreme; and we encountered all the problems most parents have, plus a few unprecedented ones. Feeding problems headed our long list, and changing formulas and schedules didn't help much. As time passed, Billy developed colic, which compounded his obvious discomfort. He was a light sleeper, day and night. It was four months before he slept through the night, and by then, both my husband and I were exhausted.

Our respite was short lived, however, for after that one night he picked up right where he left off. The least little noise awakened him, and we spent most of that first year tiptoeing about the house. What made matters worse was that he seemed to dislike being held. Most babies enjoy being warm and secure against their mother's body, but not my son. Whenever we would try to cuddle or hold him to relieve his distress or quiet his crying, he would squirm and squirm. If not released, he would stiffen his body and cry harder until he was placed back in his crib. He also disliked having anyone lean over to look at him. As anyone approached, he would start to cry again. He acted frightened.

As Billy grew older and stronger, he would wiggle constantly from one end of his crib to the other while trying to doze off. By the end of the fifth month of his life, he began to rock his crib, working himself forward until his head was hitting against the crib bumpers. The older he became, the more he rocked, the harder he banged his head, and nothing would stop him. This rocking continued, without the head-banging, until he was five years old. The only thing that gave him comfort was sucking his thumb, a habit which persisted until he was six. Then one day he just stopped doing it, by himself.

His first bath was a nerve-shattering experience for me. I slowly lowered him, cradled in my arm, into his tub and touched his toes with a few drops of water, which he accepted. As I attempted to wet him a little more, he became rigid and stopped breathing. I was so startled, I withdrew him at once and slapped him on his back. Although he resumed normal breathing in a second or two, it took me some time to stop shaking. Our later attempts were more successful, and by age two, splashing up his world was Billy's greatest pleasure.

Our son did all the physical things babies are expected to do their first year at about the appropriate time, and most things he did early. Creeping, sitting up, walking, and learning to make his needs known with simple words were not problems. The rather premature acquisition of teeth was the thing that gave him the most trouble and further complicated his eating habits. In spite of this, both his doctor and I were satisfied with his development, but I was concerned with the way he behaved.

Billy's incessant restlessness and frequent crying, for no apparent reason, disturbed me. It always lasted too long and had an abnormal intensity about it. I wouldn't say his disposition was unpleasant; instead I felt he was struggling to free himself from some strange internal stress. I could almost feel it, just watching him. His reactions to people and the world about him were unpredictable, and I often discovered that I was dealing with more than one distinct personality.

Billy looked healthy and strong, but he did not act happy or contented. He was never really calm, and I think he would have crawled out of his own skin if he could have. He seemed to strain to get away from himself, and I could not console or comfort him no matter how gently I tried. Diapering, dressing—any of the necessary ministrations—grew into a free-for-all as he gained strength. It's a wonder I never stuck him with a pin as he fought my efforts to attend his needs. Every endeavor turned into the worst hassle imaginable. He screamed and fussed outrageously, no matter how many times he had been through the same experience.

My little darling was a puzzle to me, a young and inexperienced mother. When I had first looked at him, he had reminded me of a miniature purple-faced china doll. Now, as he developed, he was the essence of an exquisite pink cherub, a beautiful child with fair skin and hair, blue eyes laced with long black lashes, and regular features. He was Dresden china personified, but his actions were incomprehensible at times.

I mentioned my feeling that all was not well with our son to my husband and my family.

"Oh, Jessie, you are a worry wart! What do you expect of him anyhow? He's just a baby and undoubtedly high strung like me," was my husband's answer. "I never saw anyone who worries about *nothing* the way you do. When I was a kid I cried a lot too." The others only laughed at me. They told me I was silly. What could you tell about a child at such a tender age? "He'll outgrow all this fussing," became a standard quotation from family and friends. Despite what anyone said, I felt there was something radically wrong with our son. Call it intuition, call me silly, but I sensed we were headed for real trouble.

By the time he was two, Billy was hyperactivity itself. At first I thought his constant moving about was due to natural childhood curiosity. He was into everything faster than I could keep up with him. I could not leave him alone for an instant. He would topple things over on himself, grab anything handy and stuff it into his mouth —always something he shouldn't have. For his safety, and to preserve my small treasures, I stripped the household of all decorative articles. China, ashtrays—

any item he could cut himself on—were removed. He had a knack for breaking ceramics that was unbelievable. Nothing escaped his attention or grasp unless it just wasn't there. He was totally incapable of sitting still, and as I looked at him moving about, it seemed to me that his motions were compulsive, as though he could not stop them himself.

One rather strange activity in which he took delight was in looking at things upside down. He not only bent himself over as far as possible to gaze at his world, but he picked up his toys and turned them upside down. If I tried to right them, he objected strenuously, and over they would go again. I kept wondering what pleasure this upside-down approach to everything gave him.

When Billy was one, he was a timid infant. When he was two, he became a fearful child. He was alarmed by almost anything. For instance? I was asked to enter his picture in a contest. The pictures were to be taken by a local department store, and the parents could select the one they liked the best as their entry. I took Billy to the photographer's studio, which had a large camera set upon a high dark-looking apparatus. After placing the child in an appropriate position and giving him some blocks to play with, the photographer began to push the dark-looking contraption slowly towards Billy. When he looked up at the approaching mechanism, he let out a scream that could have been heard two blocks away. He was in such a state of panic, it took ages to quiet him down. I was about to give up, but the photographer was persistent. All the time we tried to calm him, Billy kept looking at that camera as though it was alive and about to devour him. The man was confounded by the fear my child displayed. I guess it put a dent in his professional pride. It only worried me. In spite of the struggle, however, Billy won a prize for his photograph, tears and all.

Billy went everywhere with me, despite his increasingly abnormal and loud outbursts of distress. Some places he would not enter at all, and I had to coax him constantly. People were always offering me suggestions as to how to handle him, and strangers were always remarking on his beauty. They would gush over him, an action which he disliked immensely, and when he began to cry, they would retreat, leaving me to soothe him and try to explain his unusual behavior. Frequently I myself was stumped, trying to figure out what started him off.

I remember one particular day I took Billy grocery shopping with me. He was generally fairly well behaved if everyone left him alone. He sat in the shopping cart amusing himself with cans or packages, while I selected the items we needed. As we went down one aisle, we approached a display advertising a certain sea food. In front of the display was a mannequin dressed like a sea captain, a sort of mechanical puppet. I thought it might interest Billy, as many other young children were standing about, watching the puppet move. Halfway down the aisle, Billy looked up at this display and let out an ear-shattering scream. He grabbed me around the neck and would not let go.

"It's just a puppet, Billy, nothing to be afraid of," I explained.

"No, no, Mother, no!" was all he could say. He cried and cried, and no amount of reassuring or explaining could take away his fear. I carried him out of the store and returned that evening to complete my shopping. Afterwards, every time we came near the entrance to that or any similar store, he started to scream.

I should have saved myself the trouble of trying to talk him out of his distress—ever—for in the end he had to convince *himself* that nothing was threatening him. I could never tell in advance how Billy would react to anything or anyone at any given time. When I expected the worst, he might give me his best, and vice versa. It made life disturbingly uneasy for us. It was only by sheer determination that we managed to get anywhere or get anything done.

We found that we could not leave Billy with the most competent of baby-sitters. Either he had to come with us, or one of us had to stay at home with him. Once in a while, an occasion would arise that necessitated the presence of both of us. In this case a member of my husband's family or mine would stay with Billy. Even that was not always successful. Many times we were called home when they had trouble managing him. Such times did bring into focus all the things I had been telling them about, but everyone—especially my husband —still insisted that Billy would outgrow his peculiarities.

"You are just plain impatient," he said. "You expect Billy to be a man before he is a boy. Jessie, you have to take more time to explain things to him."

I was ready to explode. "I *do* explain things to him—" I retorted angrily. "And what do you *mean,* 'take more time'? I spend almost *all* my time with him, and he just keeps on getting upset over every trifling thing."

Our big battle had begun.

2

Daymares—Nightmares

Billy's complexities expanded to remarkable proportions as he entered his third year of life. Each part was
more upsetting to all of us than those we had previously
dealt with. He was developing into a paradox—alert,
intelligent and quick one minute; withdrawn and disturbed the next. He was always intense, even in his most
relaxed moments. The untouchable quality of internal
stress I had watched growing in him alternated with few
periods of normal calm. He seemed to be struggling un-
successfully against something. As I observed his reactions, I realized that our son was slipping into a world
of his own. It was not a world of his own making, but
one in which he was enveloped, like in a cocoon of
shadows, but from which he was unable to emerge like
the butterfly.

Often Billy did not seem to hear me when I spoke.
When he was oblivious of my speech, he was also unaware of my presence. Frequently, I had to stop him in
his activity and turn his face in my direction to make
him listen. He comprehended everything he was told,
but I found myself having to repeat certain instructions
to him before they were carried out.

During the nice weather he began to play with several
neighborhood children. As I watched him, I became

more aware that his behavior was unlike that of the others. But all the children liked Billy, and accepted him, even though he fussed one minute and was companionable the next. I know he liked them and wanted friends too, but somehow he stood apart, separated from the rest. He did develop a trust and fondness for one other child, Tommy, who lived next door. Tommy was his ally, and for years they spent a great deal of time together.

Usually the gang congregated in our yard and used Billy's toys. Billy himself displayed little interest in most of them, although he had everything imaginable. As the playing day progressed, he would lose one cherished item after another to his friends. If another child took a prized shovel or truck away from Billy, he would not fight to retrieve it. He refused to squabble with his playmates. Many times I watched him reluctantly surrender a toy to the clutches of another and become very angry —at himself.

"Billy, why don't you go after your truck?" I prodded him. "It's nice to share with others, but there are plenty of things to go around, and I know that's your favorite. Remember, if you want it, you must go after it."

He would pound his little fists against his chest in frustration instead of clouting his friend.

"I can't, I can't, I won't!" he would shout through his tears. He was completely lacking in any aggressive instincts.

It worried me that he could not stand up for himself, but constantly ran to me for help and protection. I tried to show him how to defend his right of ownership, but it was useless.

I noticed that when he was deprived of a toy, he would temporarily withdraw into his own world, dreaming, I presumed. If someone approached or disturbed him, then he would run away and cry. Basically, he was incapable of maintaining an interest in anyone very long, especially kids who annoyed him; but he was very kind to others, regardless of how they treated him. If he had a special treat of candy, cookies, or ice cream, he never failed to ask me if he could share it.

As kind and thoughtful as Billy was, he continued to dislike anyone—especially his father or me—being demonstrative towards him. It was a rare treat to be on the receiving end of a hug or kiss. Usually he refused affection with, "No, no, go away—I don't like that." He looked apprehensive if anyone came too close. He was very slow to warm up to people and particularly cautious about and shy towards strangers. However, once accepted, they were simultaneously dismissed from his attention.

Billy's lack of responsiveness to others was distressing, but something else disturbed me more. Whenever the children were outside playing, and the noonday whistle blew loud and shrill, Billy would come running into the house, screaming at the top of his lungs, his hands clasped over his ears as if he was in great pain. The first time this occurred, I thought someone had hit him, so I consoled and soothed him and sent him out to play again. When he displayed the same wild reaction to the whistle every day, I began to call him into the house for lunch early, thinking the noise just frightened him. I wondered why, as it aroused no such reactions in the others, and they continued playing without interruption. I had often seen him cringe if I raised my voice to scold or correct him, but I thought he was reacting to my anger. It never dawned on me then that his hearing was overly sensitive.

A few weeks after the first incident with the noon whistle, our son began to have nightmares. He woke up screaming at the top of his voice, and occasionally ran around the house bumping into things in the dark, in a state of confusion and bewilderment. Once in a while, we had to chase after him to subdue his thrashing, screaming torment.

"Mom! Pop! Where are you? I'm afraid!" he screamed. A dazed and shocked look contorted his face.

"Billy, Billy, it's all right. We're right here." His father would pick him up, turn on the light, and show him that all was well.

The nightmares grew steadily worse and increased in frequency. One evening after Billy had fallen asleep, I heard him talking out loud. I peeked into his room, but he was lying quietly; so I stood at his door, listening. He was talking, at the rate of a speeded-up tape recorder, about everything he had done that day. Then he woke up crying, and it was a long time before he was quiet.

As this pattern of nightmares continued, my husband and I took turns going into his room to reassure and calm him. Sometimes he hollered so long and so loud that he disturbed the neighborhood. It got so bad, we were up half the night. When Billy became afraid of the dark, we bought him a night light. For some crazy reason, he was more disturbed *with* the light than without it. Fire whistles blowing at night or stray cats serenading below his window sent him into a state of absolute panic. He often came running full speed into our room.

After months of sleepless nights and useless coaxing, we allowed him to crawl in with one of us until he relaxed. Generally, he fell asleep quickly, and we would vacate our bed and sleep in his room. I think he was nine before he had enough confidence to remain in his own room all night. Meanwhile, the game of musical beds continued.

Billy was giving me trouble at every turn of the road.

The minute the barber began to use the electric clippers on his head, he started screaming. One time he struggled so hard to free himself that the thick leather seat belt of the barber's chair snapped in two. I assume that most people watching him thought he was a spoiled brat. I could not understand why he was so afraid.

Our early feeding problems with Billy disappeared, and by age two, he was doing a splendid job of feeding himself. At age three, he refused foods he had previously enjoyed; in fact, he rejected food entirely. At first I let him go hungry, but this method did not work at all. In desperation, I gave him books to look at, toys to play with—anything to hold his attention long enough for me to get some nourishment in him. He developed strange tastes. He loved pickles and would eat anything as long as it was topped with a slice of pickle. His menus consisted of everything à la pickles—everything except milk. He drank that straight.

Naturally I consulted our pediatrician about ways and means of coping with each problem as it presented itself. He examined Billy carefully and declared there was nothing wrong with him, except that his tonsils would have to come out when he was a little older. Billy's tonsils were enormous and gave him a great deal of trouble.

One time the doctor prescribed a tranquilizer for his hyperactivity. After two doses Billy was climbing the walls. I stopped the tranquilizers immediately.

A few days after that visit to the doctor, Billy awoke one morning with his eyes swollen shut. I thought he had conjunctivitis, and was about to call the pediatrician, but my husband stopped me.

"Look, Jessie, eyes are nothing to fool around with. Take him to the best eye man in town. He may have some dirt or something stuck in there." I was sure it was nothing serious.

"But, Bill, I think it's only pink eye," I protested.

"I don't care. You do what I say," Bill insisted, as he left for work. So I called a specialist.

Billy had always been petrified by doctors, but, with careful handling, his regular visits were becoming easier. Before we kept this appointment, I informed the nurse of my son's fears so that the specialist could try to handle him with a minimum of trouble. When we arrived at his office, he sat Billy down in a chair and started to shine a flashlight in his eyes. They were inflamed and sensitive to the light, so Billy began to wiggle. The doctor grabbed my son impatiently by the shoulder and ushered him into another room. I rose to follow him, but he waved me off, saying, "Mother had better stay here."

In a few minutes I heard my son screaming, "Mother! Mother!" He sounded so distressed that I started for the door, but a nurse stopped me. She suggested that the doctor knew what he was doing, and that I should stay out! When I was allowed to enter the inner sanctum, my three-and-a-half-year-old was crimson and panting, with sweat running down his tear-soaked face. His throat was very red, too. I was furious! I wanted to get Billy out of there!

The diagnosis? Pink eye!

I took Billy to the car and slammed the door. He began to scream. Then I saw it—I had closed the door on his fingers! I pressed the handle, but the door was locked. I ran around to the other side of the car and released it. By now I was ready to faint, but I carried him into another doctor's office, and he examined the hand. No bones were broken, thank goodness!

My mother-in-law was waiting for me when I pulled

into our driveway. She took one look at me and asked, "What happened?"

As soon as I opened the door, Billy headed for his room and went to bed. He fell asleep instantly, and I removed his shirt as I talked to my mother-in-law. It was then that I saw the complete damage this "expert" had done. On my son's throat, from the base of his neck to below his ear lobes, were the long purple marks of the doctor's fingers. His ears were spotted with purple patches. His chest and upper arms were black and blue. The thing that frightened me most was a swelling on the right side of his neck.

That butcher! I thought to myself as I went for some ice. My mother-in-law headed for the phone. She told the doctor that if he did not come to the house immediately, she would call the police. He arrived within five minutes and began to shake visibly as he looked down at the sleeping child. Just then Billy opened his eyes and ran screaming from the room.

"No, no! Please, Mother, no!" he cried.

My mother-in-law took Billy in tow while I talked to the doctor. I demanded to know what had taken place behind that closed door. He said he had wrapped Billy in a sheet, to restrain him, and had placed his head between his knees in order to examine his eyes. That accounted for the bruises on his ears. What he didn't say was evident—he had lost his temper with Billy and had borne down on him so hard that he had bruised him.

I was so angry, I could have hit him. I asked him why he had not brought the child to me if he could not manage him, or at least allowed me to be present during the examination. He had no answer. He was stunned by Billy's appearance.

That night he returned to our home to apologize to my husband and son. Billy had calmed down by then, and, to the doctor's surprise, shook hands with him. The affair left its mark all the same. For a long time afterward, the word "doctor" would send Billy running from the room. It took us years to get him over his fear.

One day I was discussing Billy's peculiarities with my husband, and I mentioned that I thought our son was displaying certain characteristics of schizophrenic behavior. He exploded.

"Are you crazy? There's nothing really the matter with him. I don't think you have enough patience. Sure, he has bad moments, but so do other kids. I think you should spend more time teaching him how to manage himself, instead of complaining about what he does!" It seemed that everyone was always blaming me!

I was ready to smash Bill before he finished his tirade. My family gave me the same general response, and my father was horrified that I could entertain such a thought. Everyone conceded that Billy was a little overactive and perhaps slow to respond to instruction, but he was intelligent. I didn't dispute the fact, but I was getting sick of the same old story I kept hearing all along: "He'll outgrow all this."

Even Billy's doctor thought I exaggerated my accounts of the child's behavior. I told him often it was Billy's intensity, his unpredictability, his strange reactions to noise and normal situations that worried me. He explained in careful detail that many children rock their beds, have nightmares, suck their thumbs, and do not warm up to strangers, especially at such a young age. He said that all children are fearful at times. I kept insisting it was the degree to which Billy carried on that concerned me, but my complaints fell on deaf ears. I was condemned as an overly protective, hysterical mother. From then on, I kept my mouth shut and my thoughts to myself. Secretly, I remained anxious.

3

The Shadows Gather

"Look, *I* say he can do anything he wants to—*if* he wants to. You've seen it a thousand times! He's capable, but a loner—like I was—and that's all there is to it." My husband had *said* it a thousand times, but I still couldn't agree.

"No, that's not all there is to it," I implored. "Don't forget, he'll be starting kindergarten next year. I think we should send him to nursery school first, give him a sort of head start. He'll get used to a routine that way, and maybe he'll be more responsive to other children. He's got to learn to conform somewhere along the line, or he'll never make it in public school, Bill." How I yearned for him to agree with me.

"All right. I didn't say I was *entirely* against the idea —it just seems silly to me. However, if he's put in a position where he *has* to do more for himself, maybe he'll be less dependent." For once, Bill was almost agreeing with me! I could hardly wait to make arrangements to send our son to nursery school.

I told the school's director all about the observations I had made regarding Billy's development. She agreed to see what they could do to help prepare him for the next year.

All activities in the school were designed for fun,

learning, and social growth, and I was not surprised that Billy did not respond to any great extent. He would not sing or play with others unless he was coaxed by a teacher. For art work, he drew pictures of machines— all kinds, all shapes, and all sizes. When people were in his creations, they were always male. All his watercolors were done in purple, no matter what the subject— machines, people, sky, or grass. It took him all year to get around to riding on the playground merry-go-round, after eyeing it longingly for months.

Three times a year we received reports on Billy's progress. The first one was not encouraging. The teachers felt that nursery school was not the complete answer to his problems. They were concerned about his insecurity. When I left him in the morning, he would pace back and forth, worried that I might not return for him. Billy talked incessantly about "Jessie," but never referred to me as "mother" in his school conversations. I was surprised, because he always called me mother at home.

I told my husband about all this, and we decided to have him privately tested for I.Q. potential. Perhaps we were pushing the child beyond his abilities.

I was present when the test was administered, and the score was very low, but Billy was so distractible that I felt the score was not a true measurement of his real ability. I discussed the results of his test with his teacher. She felt, as I did, that Billy had a good deal of intelligence, but something was disturbing his capacity for functioning normally. She suggested I concentrate on getting him to do more things for himself at home.

We instituted a new regimen for Billy at once. We worked with him, getting him up a little earlier, and seeing to it that he washed, dressed, ate, and scrubbed his teeth every morning and night without help. It took forever, but we were unrelenting. Eventually, with insistence and persuasion, he got the knack of doing for himself. His biggest stumbling block was buttoning his winter coat. In the end, it was his teacher who helped him over this hurdle.

The second report reflected great improvement. Billy was more alert, responsive, and generally brighter than he had been. His insecurity had subsided, if not his hyperactivity. He did *not* improve in his relationship to other children. We constantly praised him when he did things for himself, and we continued with our home program. The minute we relaxed the gentle pressure, he began to slip backwards. His last report was distressing. The school felt Billy was intelligent and potentially capable, but they, too, were disappointed that his former progress did not continue. He was erratic, going ahead by leaps and bounds, then coming to a complete halt.

In the afternoon, after nursery school, I read to Billy a great deal. He developed an abiding love for, and a deep interest in, books. Sometimes he paid close attention when I read. When he did not, I stopped reading. My purpose was to try to capture his attention and hold it as long as possible to lessen his distractibility and stretch his attention span. Many times when I thought he was not listening, he must have been, for he could go to his bookcase and take out any book and tell you the complete story.

We also listened to records, and he learned to love music. We were never very successful at playing games —a few moments of interest, and that was it. I couldn't coax him to continue a game once he was distracted.

In further efforts to draw Billy out of his shell, we began to take him on short trips to places we felt might awaken and interest him. One trip to the Staten Island Zoo had strange results.

We entered the building which housed lions, tigers,

and other large beasts. Billy stood stark still before the Bengal tiger's cage. He watched the animal pacing back and forth for a long time, listening with rapt attention to his roaring. Billy seemed hypnotized by the tiger. Then, suddenly, he began yelling. "Shut up, I tell you, shut up!" We tried to shush him, but he would not stop. Everyone turned to see who was doing all the hollering. Billy yelled so boisterously, I wanted to melt through the concrete floor. Finally my husband picked Billy up and carried him out of the building. When his father put him down, I could see tears in the child's eyes.

I could not understand his tears at first. We had not scolded or spanked him for creating the noisy disturbance. But then I began to understand that the tears must have come from a deep feeling that the child experienced inside. He felt a spiritual kinship, unexplainable and sad, with that caged beast. His own startling outburst, after his consuming concentration on the animal's movements and sounds, was closely akin to a cry of pain!

Shortly after the zoo trip, Billy became ill with tonsillitis. He had been plagued by his large tonsils ever since he was a baby, and now his doctor said they must come out. I agreed with him, but the thoughts of sending him to the hospital threw me into a panic. However, I had no choice. How to go about preparing him—that was the monumental problem. A friend suggested I purchase a book called *A Visit to the Hospital,* and it helped enormously. We obtained the services of a doctor who was very patient and tactful. He gained Billy's confidence, a singular feat.

During a preoperative visit, while waiting for the doctor, Billy climbed up on the examining chair. There was a chart on the opposite wall, about fifteen feet away. To my surprise, my son began to read the letters on the chart out loud. I did not know he could recognize letters at all.

The tonsils were removed March 13, 1959, and I was told that Billy was an excellent patient. I was also informed that his adenoids were so large the doctor could not understand how he had breathed without difficulty. I was glad the whole thing was over.

Well, it wasn't quite over. On the 16th of March, Billy broke out with the worst case of measles imaginable. Red blobs covered him from head to toe, and he was very ill. I stayed up night and day, giving him whatever soft and soothing nourishment he could tolerate. His throat was still very sore from the tonsillectomy. As the measles spots were disappearing, I noticed a strange swelling along his jawline. Yes, he had the mumps. The succession of ailments might have floored an ordinary child, but Billy was a good patient when he was really sick. He was cooperative about taking medication, and, strangely enough, his conversations were always more lucid when he was ill than when he was well.

Although we darkened Billy's room and carefully followed the doctor's instructions while he had the measles, when he was eleven and a half years old we discovered that they had affected his sight, leaving him extremely nearsighted. Billy had never complained of poor vision. What a terrific struggle it must have been all those years, just trying to see, let alone deal with his other problems!

All through his early years, Billy's speech was normal except for frequent prolonged periods when he was very quiet. Now, quite suddenly, I noticed a marked change in his speech habits. Billy began to leave out important words of sentences. Without realizing what I was doing, I fell into the habit of supplying the missing words, and then asking him if that was what he meant. He usually said yes. I had to put snatches of conversation together like a jigsaw puzzle in order to understand him. Then too, he asked me questions constantly, a perfectly natural thing for a child, but after I answered, he repeated the same question two or three minutes later. Didn't he hear, or had he forgotten my original answer?

His talks with me were becoming maddeningly repetitious, using certain terms and phrases over and over again. I used to think his mind got hung up on one thought, and he could not proceed further. His vocabulary, which had been rather large for his age, began to diminish. Contradictory as it may sound, his intellectual curiosity was beyond his years. He would talk about atomic powered submarines, radio or television antennas and the necessity for them, thermometers and what they measured, and manual gear shifts as opposed to automatic shifts for automobiles and trucks. Mechanical devices of all kinds fascinated him.

I noticed a change in Billy's eating habits too.

When he was three, he had rejected many foods for a while, but later had resumed eating almost everything. Now, once again, he began rejecting almost everything eatable. He could not abide the smell or taste of former favorites, *especially* pickles. I tried to vary his diet as much as possible within his rapidly diminishing preferences.

In addition to these changes in speech and eating habits, Billy's walking pattern began to fluctuate, from his formerly smooth rhythm to movements strange to behold. At times his gait looked odd, as though he was about to stumble and was struggling to recover his balance. Billy was never a clumsy child, and had displayed remarkable balancing ability at an early age, but now he frequently looked awkward.

The more I observed Billy's crazy growth and regression patterns, the more convinced I became that something was wrong with him. My fears were somewhat allayed after nursery school, during the summer vacation which we spent at the shore. Some of Billy's oddities disappeared, but not for long. In the meantime, my family and I kept running around the same old tree.

"He is growing out of all this; he is coming along. Just give him a chance," they said. But I carried a lump of anxiety around inside me. It refused to untangle, especially as we neared the start of Billy's first year in kindergarten.

I had taken time, after our vacation, to walk with our son to the neighborhood school he would be attending in September, 1959. I talked to him about his behavior, and how he was growing up, and what would be expected of him in class. He seemed to understand. Perhaps public school would stimulate a change in him for the better.

The first day, as we were greeted by his teacher, I relaxed to see that Billy was pleased with his new surroundings. He had been in school about three weeks when I was called for a conference with his teacher. Her obvious dislike for me and my child was hardly masked as we talked. She told me that Billy was "just not with it." His actions were disruptive to the class, she said. Apparently he was bothering the life out of her. She told me she had never seen such a "different" child. I think, if she had had the authority, she would have thrown both of us out, right then and there. I found out later, from my aunt who taught in the same school, that my son had spent most of those first three weeks sitting in the principal's office, being completely ignored by everyone. I wondered how he could have been so intolerable to his teacher if he had been absent from her classroom most of the time.

Following the interview with the teacher, my husband and I were called into the school psychologist's office. He said that Billy had been tested, and he felt our son was too immature to be attending school at this time, even though he was five and a half. He also said he had a trained eye and could "spot one of these children by just looking through the classroom door."

"What do you mean by 'one of these' children?" I asked. "Do you mean to imply that you are assuming that Billy is retarded, on the basis of *one test?*" He did not reply, so I went on. "Well, we are his parents, and we know him better than you do." He did not argue with that, and my husband continued.

"What were the scores on the I.Q. test you administered to Billy?" Bill asked. The psychologist answered him indirectly, implying that his score was between 70 and 80, indicating a very low mentality.

When we thought of Billy's interests and the advanced subjects he often discussed at home, we were stunned. I didn't care what measurement they had used! I did not believe it was accurate, and neither did my husband.

The psychologist's conclusions were that we should not expect much of our child, who was obviously retarded. If he behaved well, he would be allowed to continue in regular school; if not, he would have to attend a special school. Aside from his theory of retardation, the psychologist told us that the strange emotional problems Billy displayed were caused by the way we had treated him from birth. About now I was coming to a slow boil. *What gall!* I fumed. *What made him think he knew how we had treated our son?* The meeting had one dramatically good effect. My husband finally realized that I was *not* an overanxious mother, and that we had to do something to help our son. Once aroused, he was stirred to action.

Our third interview took place the next day in the office of the school principal. He was a dour man, and his attitudes cloaked me like a blanket of gloom and doom. The consensus of the teacher, the psychologist, and the principal was that Billy was relatively hopeless, but that we should get professional help for him if we could afford it. We were not told to remove him from kindergarten, but after all the interviews, it was obvious to us that Billy would be pushed aside and ignored if we allowed him to continue. We decided to withdraw him and try again another year.

When we told our son, as gently as possible, that he would not be going back to class, he was bewildered and disappointed, thinking he had done something wrong. He could not understand why he had been taken out of school. It hurt us so much to watch his unhappiness, that we enrolled him in another nursery school.

In the meantime, the way was clearly marked. My husband knew, now, that we must get help for Billy and find the cause of his emotional instability and strange development patterns. He contacted a psychiatrist of good reputation and gave him all the information he could about Billy's personality and growth. After examining our son, he told us that Billy was definitely *not* retarded, but was suffering from a severe emotional disturbance. He suggested we have him neurologically evaluated and clinically tested for I.Q. potential, using a method different from that used by the school where he had been enrolled. He said we should take advantage of the facilities of the local mental health clinic, because treatment for Billy might be long and expensive. As director of the Clinic, he would keep close watch over Billy's progress.

Bill and I immediately made appointments for neurological and I.Q. testing, and we went to the clinic's psychiatric social worker to hear the results. He greeted us glumly, took out his pocket watch, wound it, and set it on the desk in front of him. This struck me as rather odd, for there was a clock on the wall he could have referred to by merely turning his head. For the next fifty minutes he related to us the results of the neurological examination and the I.Q. test, which showed Billy to have normal or above average intelligence and severe emotional problems, which I had suspected for years. The psychiatrist entered our son's name on a waiting list, and said we would be hearing from him soon. With this summation we were dismissed.

Meanwhile, Billy wasted another year going to nursery school for the second time. His attitude of "take it or leave it" toward others continued, and now he began to verbalize imaginative fantasies continuously. When I listened carefully, I saw that they reflected his internal anxieties and conflicts. Talking about them out loud was an effort on his part to allay his ever-mounting fears. He still worried that I would not return for him at school, but when I did, I was usually ignored. He still had nightmares, but they were fewer and shorter. His hyperactivity was ever with him.

The woman in charge of his school often remarked about Billy's "mental static." To her, he acted as if he had loose wires in his head, and when they touched, he became disturbed. At other times, he was as normal and helpful as the other children.

I remember one incident of helpfulness that bordered on old-fashioned mischief. Billy stayed with my two aunts one night when my husband I were busy elsewhere. The next morning he got up early to explore their apartment. They didn't hear him making much noise, so they assumed he was drawing or looking at a book, and they did not bother to get up and check on him right away. It was an expensive mistake.

My aunts had recently purchased a chair for the living room. It was covered in a nylon fabric, trimmed about the arms, back, and bottom with fringe. Billy had never seen a chair like it, and the fringe must have looked inappropriate to him. When my aunts decided to get up and see what he was doing, they walked into the living room and nearly fell over. There was our son, scissors in hand, giving the chair a fringe-cut. Luxurious trim was strewn all about as he went industriously about his work. Needless to say, they were a bit upset, but, fortunately, our insurance covered the cost of having the chair reupholstered. Billy was forgiven.

About the same time as the chair-trimming incident, I saw a peculiar phenomenon take place in Billy every now and then. He would be sitting in a chair, looking at a book, and suddenly his face would change color. He went from rosy-cheeked health to a deathly white pallor in a few seconds. This was often followed by outbursts of crying and fussing. It happened frequently just before mealtime, and Billy would not calm down until after he had eaten. I mentioned this color change to the doctor, and he had Billy's blood tested. The results showed nothing physically wrong. I asked myself a million times if this was really true. Why, then, was he having such great difficulty functioning? Why was he emotionally disturbed? Why did the way he acted and looked at times contradict all the different doctors' reports? No one ever gave me a satisfactory answer so we kept boxing shadows.

At age six Billy was capable of caring for his physical necessities, but he was ever a reluctant dragon. He insisted on maintaining a dependent relationship with anyone who would do things for him. His father and I tried perpetually to lead him into a more independent attitude, but he would have none of it. When I refused to help him, he would be incensed. Only when he ardently desired to do something would he take the initiative. If he did accomplish some feat, he was generally astonished by his own success.

Although Billy had been riding his two-wheeled bicycle for some time with helping wheels attached, he refused to let his father remove the training wheels. Despite the fact that most of the time they were off the ground as he rode, he would not agree to give them up. Ignoring his protestations, his father removed first one wheel and, about a week later, the other. He gave Billy a shove, and away he went, looking back every once in a while, hardly believing he was riding with just two wheels. This sort of negative approach to trying anything new, this reluctance to trust himself, impeded him tremendously. We found, however, that with encouragement and guidance eventually he would do well. We hoped our helping him along would carry over to a more successful school year.

4

The Disturbing, the Good, the Bad

Once more our son attended the school he had gone to briefly the previous year. This time he was in a different classroom, with a different teacher. At the same time, he began psycho-play therapy once a week as a patient of the local mental health clinic. While Billy was with his psychiatrist, I spent the hour talking to a social worker. He wanted to know my life's history, starting as far back as I could remember. I thought this was ridiculous, but I wanted to help Billy, so I tried to answer the man's questions as truthfully as possible. When he persisted in asking me very personal questions about my relationship with my husband, I became more than angry. I did not consider my bedroom affairs a suitable topic for discussion. One day he remarked to me that I seemed to walk mentally around the obstacles he kept placing in my path.

My husband went through the same third degree, and when the same social worker started to zero in on him with prying, he lost his temper. He told the man it was "none of his damn business." At one point they nearly came to blows. Bill was never loquacious about his deepest feelings or concerns to anyone, not even to me. Oh, he talked about Billy, but what he truly felt at this time,

I never knew. I did know what he felt about the social worker, however.

"That damned numbskull!" Bill sputtered. "I absolutely refuse to spend any more time with him! Besides, I don't know how much longer they'll allow me to take an hour off each week. I don't think my boss appreciates it, and I don't blame him. Will you please tell me what that guy is aiming at anyhow? What good is all this dribble doing Billy?" My husband was furious.

"I can't see much sense to it all myself, Bill," I agreed, "but if it helps Billy, it's worth it. I wish you wouldn't get so angry about it."

I tried to console him, but he remained unsoothed. I agreed with him on one point. I didn't see what all this palaver about our own lives had to do with our son's situation. We were responsible adults. We did not abuse our son. But somehow we both got the impression that the social worker thought we were misguided idiots. It was infuriating, and I, for one, resented his attitude tremendously. After all, we had come this far in life without his particular brand of invisible "help."

Four or five months passed, and Bill and I asked to have a joint conference with the social worker and the psychiatrist. At the meeting we plied them with questions. As usual we received no answers of consequence. We wanted to know the exact nature of Billy's problem, but they would not put a name tag on it.

Instead of delving deeply into the purpose of the meeting, the psychiatrist wanted to know if Billy was receiving religious instruction. When she asked us this, I was dumbfounded. One of us asked her why she wanted to know. She told us that somehow Billy was preoccupied with a fear of the devil. It took me a few seconds to realize what she was getting at and then we both almost burst out laughing. Sometimes I used a canned lunchmeat. On the can there was a small picture of a devil. I remember Billy asking me what that creature was. "It's a devil, Billy," I told him. "Why do you ask?"

"Because it has a tail and horns and it looks funny," was all he replied. We dropped the conversation there.

Religious instruction indeed!

For an hour our talk continued, everyone bouncing words about, without anyone wanting to catch the verbal ball. I could sense my husband's impatience growing along with my own. He is an intelligent and direct man, always going right to the heart of the problem, and this pointless discussion was getting on his nerves. Mine too. The sum and substance of the meeting boiled down to the advice that we should work as a team for our son's benefit. What did they think we were trying to do already? There was no explicit information given us concerning Billy's troubles or their source. We learned nothing new. We were disgusted. We wanted information, suggestions—anything we could use to alleviate the child's vacillating emotional disorder. Talk about frustration! It was so thick I could have bitten it! That is how our meeting ended, with two apparently satisfied professionals and two still-anxious parents.

On the way home, my husband had some comments to make about using the team approach to a problem. He had been a B-17 pilot during World War II, with hours of combat duty over Germany to his credit. His very life and the lives of others had depended on team work. Each man on the team knew what was expected of him. Each one did his part to insure success for all in the end.

"How can we help him if they don't tell us what ails him?" Bill complained. "I tell you, Jessie, this is the craziest team approach to his troubles I have ever had the misfortune to be involved in. If they can't trust us with the diagnosis, we've been eliminated from their team before the game has started!" He was utterly exasperated.

Although our conference was unrewarding, Billy was benefiting from his therapy. One unexpected dividend he derived from his psycho-play activities was that of learning to express his feelings by drawing. He drew pictures constantly, pictures in the manner of Van Gogh, full of motion, chaos and violence, carefully detailed. He drew mechanical things as he had in nursery school, from every angle, even from above the subject, looking down on it. His terrifying emotions and his restlessness could be felt, just by looking at his handiwork. His art was explosive in concept. He kept on drawing for years until he later switched to writing imaginative stories. I could have papered a couple of houses with his artistic endeavors. My brother-in-law supplied us with drawing paper, or we would have been bankrupt.

Unhappily, Billy did *not* improve in his relationship to others in school. I was glad that he had his pal, Tommy. Tommy appointed himself Billy's protector and defender, and they were always together, though they were in different classes. Tom boosted Billy's courage more than once. That helped. He was also Billy's "hurry up-er," for Billy was ever "Slow Man on the Totem Pole," a study in suspended animation.

His report card reflected his difficulties, and his teacher told me that he seemed nervous, but happy, in the group. At the end of the year, she wrote us that Billy would be promoted on a probationary basis, because most first grade work depended on participation in reading and other groups. She commented on my son's kindness and how hard he tried to overcome his fears.

Pacing like the caged tiger became a habit with Billy.

Stress of any sort would trigger it off. The more worried he became, the faster he would stride back and forth, always on the balls of his feet. When it came time to face an issue, however, he sometimes mustered enough self-control to get through the ordeal. I remember how he behaved when confronted with the unpleasant, but necessary, removal of a plantar wart from his right foot.

Each night we applied medication to the wart, and after a week, we went to the doctor to have the destroyed part taken off. Billy paced up and down, making me dizzy watching him, until his turn came. In the office, he lay quietly as the doctor carefully cut away with his scalpel. I used to think that I could not have held still for this treatment. I was constantly amazed by Billy's courage and his contradictory obsessive fears.

He finally finished kindergarten, for the third year in a row, while going to the clinic for therapy each week. We were told that when he entered first grade, there would be no time available for his appointments with the psychiatrist, except during school hours. His father and I felt this would be too disruptive, and, since he had not shown too much improvement, we decided to struggle on alone and see how matters went. We were looking forward to a pleasant summer, when our plans were changed by a series of unforeseen events.

First we found out that I had to have major surgery immediately. As I was recovering, my mother-in-law's health began to fail. She had suffered with heart trouble for years but her condition suddenly deteriorated. We thought we would lose her. My own father died first, of a heart attack on August 14. She followed him to the grave on September 16. It was a sad time for all of us, and our son felt their loss deeply; how deeply, I did not know right away.

We did not allow him to attend their funerals, but he

did ask to see their graves. He placed a few flowers near the headstones, and began to ask about where his grandparents had gone. When I asked him if he knew the answer to his own question, he quickly replied, "Oh, yes. Their bodies are in the ground, but their souls are in Heaven with God." Then he asked us to leave him alone at the gravesites. We walked some distance away, and when I looked back, my son was kneeling on the ground, his little hands clasped together, his face turned up to the sky. He was praying for his grandparents' immortal souls to rest peacefully forever.

Later he asked me if I thought they had heard him. I assured him they had, and told him they would be happy to know how much he had loved them both.

The terrible summer gone, we turned our attention to Billy's progress in the first grade. It could be called a relatively quiet year. He learned to read, write, and do arithmetic; but he continued living in his private world, unaffected by the presence of others. He made just one attempt to wiggle his way out of it, again in a curious fashion. Because he wished to communicate and did not know how to go about it, or because he desired attention from his peers, Billy kept pretending he was a machine. Every day the children would ask him what he was. It got to be a game. He would reply that he was a steam roller, a front-end loader, an engine, or what have you. When I found out what he was doing, I told him repeatedly that he was a fine boy, and we loved him —that he was not a machine. Weeks later he gave up pretending.

Billy's hyperactivity quieted down, and so did his conversations with me. The only way I knew what was going on in school was by asking the teacher. She really liked Billy, and was kind and patient with him. She told me he was a very good reader. He did well in language, music and art, but he was only fair at arithmetic. His report card reflected his gains, and even his social habits were passable, a tremendous improvement over preceding years.

"You know, I am really enchanted by your son. Did you know what a sense of humor he has?" she asked me one day.

"That is a trait I have never seen him display at home," I confessed.

"Well, the other day I had all the children outside for gym, and while we were playing a game, I accidentally tripped one of my students. Billy came over, looked me in the face with a very serious expression and said, 'You're fired!' Then he burst out laughing. He was teasing me," she explained.

I was beginning to feel hopeful that our boy was changing for the better. He ceased the repetitive questioning in which he had engaged before, but now he became forgetful. If it rained, and he wore overshoes to school, he would walk home without them. I despaired of trying to get him to remember scarves, gloves, and other paraphernalia, but I knew this kind of forgetting wasn't uncommon for his age. The worrisome thing was the way he looked at me when I asked him what had happened to his possessions. He was a complete blank; he didn't know what I was talking about.

The year rolled on, and we noticed Billy's general approach to schoolwork had an unusual quality about it. He worried himself from step to step. He lacked flexibility in his learning patterns and personality traits. He was slowly becoming very rigid and set in his ways. He experienced difficulty in making the transition from one learning situation to another, invariably struggling through a short period of agitation. Once he understood a concept, however, he rarely forgot it, for he had a phenomenal memory.

Never enthusiastic about participating in sports or games, Billy *did* enjoy watching golf and bowling matches on television. His father spent hours trying to teach him how to play baseball, badminton—any game he thought he could enjoy with other boys. As I watched them, I could not understand why Billy ducked or ran away every time his father threw a ball in his direction. He seemed to be afraid of being hurt, or at least that is the way it looked then. He would not go down a hill on his sled either, unless his dad or I held him on. Considering all this, we enrolled him at the local Y.M.C.A. We hoped it might stir an athletic spark in him.

Billy took to swimming like a young fish. He had only one problem at the Y. He was slow, slow, slow. Everyone kept hurrying him.

At the end of the Y.M.C.A. season, Billy took part in an athletic circus. It was a pleasing and rare moment, watching him perform gymnastic feats. He enjoyed the activities so much we sent him to the Y summer camp. We thought it would be fun for him and help him to think for himself more, breaking his dependence on us for companionship. He did fairly well, but after strenuous morning fun he complained of excessive fatigue. After he had eaten lunch and rested, the fatigue was less troublesome.

His first grade year was busy. Besides his regular school and Y.M.C.A. sessions, Billy attended religious training classes once a week, after regular school hours. He had been baptised in his father's religion, and for a number of years, went to Sunday Mass with him. He did not understand the ritual but seemed to get comfort from going to the services. Now he had prayers to learn, and he asked me searching questions about the Bible. I bought him a book of Bible stories and read it to him. When we were reading together from the Gospel, he would ask me very deep and interesting questions. More than once he asked me what God looked like, and if He was really there, why did He allow people to be sick or unhappy?

"Why can't we touch God?" Billy asked me. I was impressed with his depth of understanding. Some questions were impossible to answer, so I told him we just had to accept certain things as being true, that this was known as having faith.

First grade was a good year, although certain symptoms Billy had displayed since birth persisted. We hoped the trend he was showing would continue. Perhaps he might outgrow his poor start.

I was soon to realize that first grade was but an interlude of peace in our sea of turmoil.

5

Problems and a Diagnosis

Two months of second grade had disappeared before Billy's new battle began. The children started to tease him because of the way he behaved, and, I suppose, because he ignored them when they spoke to him. As a result of the teasing, he began to have temper tantrums, sometimes four, five, or more a day—screaming, thrashing, explosions! His pal, Tommy, had to sit on him to help him calm down on the way home from school. He became so frustrated trying to deal with their constant harassment, that he came home upset and crying every day at lunchtime. It was a daily occurrence for me to soothe his distress, feed him, and see if I could straighten out whatever had shaken him up that day. Habitually, the oil I poured on troubled waters did the trick. I could successfully talk him out of his disturbance. I wondered how he managed to do his school work at all some days.

I attempted to talk to his teacher about the teasing but she always seemed to be just leaving school, or had a previous appointment, or some other excuse. Finally, I went to the principal, and he spoke to her about the teasing. She bluntly told him there was very little she could do to control it. As for Billy, it was obvious she considered him a pain in the neck, and wasn't going to waste much time on him. I thought her attitude as a professional teacher was shameful. I wasn't asking her for much, just to keep an eye out for trouble while he was in her class. With her cooperation, we might be able to make things go better for Billy.

Most of the time, my heart was in my throat when lunchtime rolled around. Often I walked over to meet Billy. I never knew in what state he would arrive, or what would happen next. I walked a tightrope of anxiety.

In spite of the daily abuse he took from others, I had never heard him say he disliked or hated another child. He never gave up trying to get along, and Tommy, his ever present help in time of trouble, would fight anyone he saw bullying Billy or taunting him. At times Billy would express dismay at being teased. He did not understand why some of the children poked fun at him and called him stupid. Many others liked Billy, but expressed concern to me that he was so afraid of everything and everybody.

One afternoon after school, Billy came running home, violently aggravated. He passed me like a shot, headed for his room, and began to tear it apart. He threw his books, records, and toys all over the room. Anything and everything went flying. I ran after him and stopped him, just as he was about to topple his dresser over. He had the strength of a demon, and all the pent-up frustration he had suffered for months came to the surface. He screamed and cried. A flood of hostility for the world and everyone in it, including his parents, poured forth like water rushing past a collapsing dam.

"I hate them! I hate them! I hate you and everyone!" I couldn't believe my ears as he violently expressed his terrible state of mind.

All of a sudden, Billy ran to me and threw his arms around my neck, squeezing with all his might. He sobbed for more than an hour as I held him in my arms. I thought his little heart was permanently broken. He begged to know why nobody liked him, or wanted to be his friend, or helped him, and why he was so unhappy. As I listened to him, I prayed, "My God, my God, he's so young. Have pity on him, and show me the way to help my precious child."

When the storm finally passed, we put his room back in order, talking quietly as we worked. I tried to explain that to be a friend, we have to take an interest in other people. We cannot expect them to care for us if we do not care for them. I know he did not completely understand my meaning, but for a long time after the torrent, Billy was calmer.

Often, as we talked together, especially after such an upsetting day, I watched something that was difficult to explain. I would see another child in him, as if a curtain parted, and there, behind the shadows of distress, the incessant turmoil, and the confusion, was an intelligent, sensitive, normal, thinking human being. If only others knew him as I did! How gentle and kind he really was! How painful it was for us, watching him fighting for a place in life, not being able to do more to ease his way.

When we witnessed this overwhelming force slowly destroying Billy's ability to function, my husband said, "You know, he acts as if he is cycling in his behavior."

"What do you mean, cycling?" I asked him.

"It's hard to describe," Bill acknowledged, "but he acts as if there is too much adrenalin pouring into him sometimes. You know, it fires him up."

The nail had been hit on the head, but, in our ignorance, we were missing the point.

Chaos continued, and Billy's general reluctance to do

things for himself came to a head in gym class. Shoe tying had always bugged him, but he had become perfectly capable of performing the task. Now he was unable to do it, no matter how many times I showed him. As we practiced the art, he fumbled around like a child making his first attempts. In school, his teacher just let him struggle until, in sheer desperation, Billy once again taught himself how to do it. I could not figure out how he could have had such an everyday skill and lose it. There were other things he had known how to do for years that he forgot completely. I had to reteach him. It was puzzling. In other matters he was unchangeable.

One morning, for instance, he went next door to pick up his pal for school, but Tom was sick. Instead of knocking and, after a short interval, going on his way, he knocked so hard he broke the glass storm door. I asked him later why he didn't just go on. "But I always go with Tommy," was his answer. Once he had established a routine, he saw no necessity for changing it—glass doors, sick friends, or anything else notwithstanding.

I was happy that Tommy stuck close to Billy, and when they were not involved in other activities, they played together in our cellar. They built all sorts of things out of old boxes, chairs—any and all available materials. As they played, Billy transposed his fantasies into action. They stuffed old clothes with newspapers to make people. They painted, puttered, drew—always together. Tommy often told me Billy had the *best* ideas. I think he meant that Billy had a strange and wild imagination.

Billy's playing ways were vastly different from Tommy's, and he was unbending in his insistence on doing things his way. Tom was just as insistent on his. If they came to an impasse of wills or ideas, I had to step in and redirect their attention to something new, getting their minds away from the controversy. Only once did Billy really get annoyed with Tommy. Then he picked him up by the seat of his pants and the back of his neck and literally threw him out the back door. Tommy just came back in by the front door. They made me laugh. They made a more amusing team than Laurel and Hardy. In spite of flying sparks, Billy liked to have his friend come to his house to play. This suited me, for I could keep an eye on them and step in if necessary.

One day they decided to make a jail out of an old playpen. Billy was the prisoner, Tommy the sheriff. Billy crawled inside the upside down playpen, looked around, and began to scream, although no one was near him. Upstairs, I thought he was hurt, and I ran down the flight of steps and tried to pull him out. He looked paralyzed with fear and wouldn't—or couldn't—budge. Finally, Tommy and I lifted the make-believe prison off him. Extricated at last, he was shaking with fright. Moments such as this rattled me. I could not figure out what instigated his terror.

About then, Billy learned to play chess. His father taught him the game, and he was very good at it. He even asked for a book to explain the game further. I mused on his terrible inconsistency. It was not that other children were not inconsistent, or didn't have setbacks at different stages of growth, but Billy did everything to such extremes!

Having to relearn to tie his shoes, being frightened out of his wits by a playpen, and then learning a game difficult even for adults—none of it made sense. Ours was a cockeyed household, to say the least.

Billy's report cards reflected this crazy design too. Scholastically, his work was satisfactory, but the conduct side of his report card was terrible. He did not listen attentively, complete his work on time, exercise self-control, or work well with others. But somehow he managed to get through second grade and survive it all.

That summer we took him to visit relatives in Massachusetts. He had two uncles—identical twins—two aunts, and three male cousins. A fourth male cousin was added years later. Both uncles were newspapermen, and one owned a farm with two horses. Billy enjoyed feeding them, and his uncle managed to get him on one of the horses for a ride.

Billy liked everything about the farm and delighted in riding around it in an old broken-down truck driven by one of his older cousins. I could actually see him relax a little. He was happy; but then he usually was, with his own. It was the outside world that frightened him. He could not deal with it except in a very awkward and restrictive way. His cousins were aware of this "difference" and called him "little Billy," although he was bigger than the cousin his age. They were kind and understanding if he became negative. Billy unconsciously responded to this innately sympathetic feeling they had for him.

From Massachusetts we drove to Mystic, Connecticut, and New London. My husband had a pass from his reserve service, so we were allowed on the submarine base there.

Billy was intrigued by the ships, but at close inspection, they overwhelmed him. He began to tremble visibly as we walked along the docks, looking at one dark hull after another. We had no such reaction from him at Mystic, where he was very interested in looking at the boats formerly owned by famous people. He kept asking me how a crippled man had managed to sail his boat. I explained that many people have handicaps and, with some help, are able to overcome them. I know what I said hit home, as he gave me a long intense look as I spoke to him.

We took our son everywhere we went, and, no matter how disruptive he became, or how upset, we did not try to hide him. I became immune to people's questioning glances and remarks when he fussed or hollered. We did not care what anyone thought, and our vacation was very successful. But September was upon us. Once again we had to boost Billy's courage and ready him for another school year.

Starting with review of the previous year's work, he had little trouble. He had a marvelous memory, and his mind had retained what he had learned before. When the new work was presented, however, he bogged down again, and it became necessary for us to support his efforts.

Toward the middle of third grade, Billy was having great difficulty with arithmetic assignments. His attention span, which was already short, decreased. When he worked, he erased constantly, refusing to hand in a paper unless he felt it was absolutely perfect. This slowed him down to a crawl, and things went from bad to worse in class.

Billy kept bringing his books home, but he never knew what his homework was. We had to call others to find out. His teacher told me he would come to school in the morning, look at his assigned work on the board, and be overwhelmed.

"I know from his past records that his capabilities are very low, so I try not to push him too hard." She was trying to be helpful.

But I became angry. After all, we had spent a great deal of money having Billy privately tested, and his problem was *not* lack of ability. I explained all this to the teacher. She looked at me as though I was crazy.

"Do you think it would help him if we engaged a tutor, especially in arithmetic?" I asked, determined not to let him fall behind.

"No, but if you could help him at home I think it would be beneficial," she suggested.

From then on we supervised Billy's work, and his father drilled him on the multiplication tables until he knew them perfectly. With our help, he crawled out of the scholastic mire into which he was rapidly sinking. Working with him, we realized, however, that his problem was not getting better. If he was relaxed, he could absorb knowledge quickly, and knew exactly what it was all about. Another time, he would fade behind a wall. We could not penetrate his dark retreat.

We helped him all we could that year, but had many arguments about it. We tried not to discuss our frustrations in front of him, but, like all children, he had big ears if we tried to talk privately. We both found it difficult to keep quiet when we should have.

I felt we were supporting him too much, and that he would lose the small initiative he did have. His father felt he needed help in order to make any progress; otherwise, he would become hopelessly lost and befuddled. Actually, we were both right. I kept asking myself, "Billy, Billy, Billy, why are we having such a terrible time raising you?" But no one answered my question.

The coldest part of the winter was gone when I decided to allow Billy to ride his bicycle to school. If he was to learn to move out on his own, he would have to start sometime. I could not follow him about forever, protecting him against life. A couple of times he walked home at noon, forgetting that his bike was at school. I shall never forget one day when he came running into the house, all upset and crying. Through his tears, he told me that some big boy had taken his bicycle by force and repeatedly laughed at him, calling him "stupid," plus a few other choice names.

"I am *not* stupid, Mother, I am *not!*" he cried out to me.

I agreed, and while he ate lunch, I took the car and searched for the lost bike. I found it about two blocks away, but never did learn which boy took it. The temporary loss of the bicycle did not upset me. But I *was* upset by the way the boy's words wounded my son.

Despite this incident and an occasional brush with some kids at school, Billy *did* seem more aware of the presence of others that year. He found another friend too, a boy named Michael.

Billy and his new friend were invited down to the next block to play one afternoon. It was the first time I could remember Billy's wanting to go to another place to play. I was happy that, at last, he was reaching out beyond the confines of home to seek companionship. It was still cold when the two boys, warmly dressed, took off on their bicycles. They had been gone about half an hour when I heard Billy screaming horribly. I ran to the back door to see what was the matter.

Billy was riding up on his bicycle at full speed, his face scarlet, dirty, and tear-soaked. His scarf, coat, gloves, and hat were missing. I ran toward him, and he fell into my arms, crying and screaming over and over, "They don't like me, Mother! Oh, why don't they like me?" His question was full of anguish.

I tried to find out what had happened, and through his sobbing, he told me that the boys had taken his clothes and poked fun at him, all the while calling him names, tormenting him with teasing. They had ganged up on him and Michael. The whole invitation had been a trick to get the two boys alone. At this point I did not know what to say.

"Billy, Billy, please don't cry." I tried to console him. "No matter what anybody else says or does, you know we love you. So do your friends, Tommy and Michael. I'm sorry that not everyone is kind."

I felt so sick for him the tears began to roll down my own face. When Billy saw that I was crying too, he tried to console *me*. He suddenly became very calm, and, with remarkable poise, looked at me and said, "It's all right, Mom. I can stand it."

Then I really lost control and began to sob. It killed me to know that this child, who wanted friendship and understanding so desperately, had been completely rejected, and there was nothing I could do about it.

We both composed ourselves, and I took Billy back to collect his missing clothing. The offending boys were still there, standing around looking ashamed. I did not ask them why they had treated the two boys so badly. I said nothing at all. What good would it have done?

Billy never went away from the house to play after this experience, but he forgot the hurt they had inflicted on him. It took me a great deal longer to be forgiving.

The school year was drawing to a close, and his father and I grew increasingly concerned about our son's dependence on us for help with his school work. The psychologist with whom we had originally dealt was no longer with the school system. A new man had taken his place. We decided to get in touch with him and have a talk about Billy and his learning disabilities, as well as his poor adjustment. The hours we had spent helping him all year should have had more fruitful results.

Up to this time, we had been working in the dark—except for my private opinion—regarding the exact nature of Billy's emotional disability. It was not until this appointment in June, 1963, that we were finally told the truth.

We gave written permission for the new psychologist to obtain the original diagnosis, made years before at the local mental health clinic. When we kept our appointment, he read us the document. The diagnosis was childhood schizophrenia, the prognosis guarded. I looked at my husband as the psychologist read the findings to us. He looked apologetic. Something inside me screamed in pain. I knew it! I knew it! When I thought of how the boy was suffering, I felt sick at my stomach. It was like hearing the death knell sounded. I felt even worse, realizing that this original diagnosis had been made when the child was six, and here we were, hearing the truth three and a half years later! Had we known sooner, perhaps we could have done more to help him.

I appreciated the man's honesty, but when he inferred that the psychological damage had been done by the way we handled Billy in the first five years of his life, I burned. What did he imagine we had done to him?

In the next breath, the psychologist told us that Billy was intelligent, but that we should get out of his education and leave the teaching to his teachers. My blood pressure rose. What did he think the purpose of this meeting had been? What did he think we had been trying to do? It was no pleasure to spend hours trying to straighten out our son's misery and confusion over his work. We had been attempting to do at home what nobody seemed to be able to do in school. He urged us to seek further psychotherapy for Billy.

"What are you so upset about, Jessie?" Bill asked me. "He's still the same boy we've always had. Nothing has changed." I knew my husband was right, but I was crushed.

After the meeting, I contacted the psychiatrist who had examined Billy originally and asked if he could take our son as a private patient. I filled him in on everything we had observed about Billy in the intervening years, and he agreed to start working with him in September, 1963.

Billy asked us if we would have someone help him a little with arithmetic that summer. We thought it would give him an edge for the fourth grade. It wasn't much—half an hour, twice a week for four weeks. We saw to it that he had plenty of recreation too. We bought a large portable pool for the yard, and he and the neighborhood children spent hours swimming and fooling around in it. The Y.M.C.A. had helped develop his swimming ability, and his general physical prowess grew. I sensed a little budding self-confidence as he showed off, swimming with his friends.

We did everything we could think of to help him grow up and be happy. Meanwhile, we hoped he would improve when he started psychotherapy in the fall. We kept trying to change him in spite of the finality, the hopelessness, of that awful diagnosis.

To us, Billy was a diamond in the rough. Held to the light, the stone looked very cloudy, but we knew the potential was there. How to cut the facets and release its inner brilliance—that was the great problem.

6

Uphill—Downhill

Our son's character was ever growing, not for the better, not entirely for the worst. The war that raged within him sent him in countless directions at one and the same time. The incidence of normal and abnormal reactions to his surroundings and to people increased rapidly. On the one hand, he progressed, on the other, he didn't. A contradictory state of affairs was acceptable fare for Billy. Each day those of us who were closest to him—his father, myself, his teacher, and his psychiatrist—were presented with another aspect of Billy's internal conflict. This year marked the greatest maturity we had witnessed in him so far, and simultaneously, the start of a long downhill slide.

The first two months of school sailed by smoothly, but, once again, as new work was presented, we all were ensnared in a scholastic trap. To keep Billy in stride with the class, we had to step in and help, especially with arithmetic. Often, if he did not get something clearly during the morning hours of school, he would bring the work home at noon. While he ate lunch, I would do my best to sort out his confusion and work with him until he got things straight. He always knew when he was not grasping the substance of a lesson, and he could not settle for less than absolute perfection. He was his own severest critic.

As I guided him through the rough spots, I kept thinking about the school psychologist's words, "Leave the teaching to the teacher." How we wished we could! But when we withdrew our support, Billy fell flat on his face, and his emotional problems swelled with the rising tide of fear of failure, until he was immobilized by their force.

Bill and I talked again about getting a tutor to help him, but my husband was an expert in math, and he couldn't accept this solution.

"I know the child, Jessie," he argued, "and I see how to approach him to get the point across. I see where his weaknesses are. I can teach him." Bill was supremely confident that he could handle the situation.

The school psychologist had implied to us that if we had Billy tutored, he would feel pushed beyond his capabilities. We were left in a quandary—condemned if we did, caught if we did not. We did the best we could. It was never good enough.

Billy told me many times that he found it difficult to keep his thoughts on what he was doing. He said he caught himself daydreaming in class constantly, and forgot what was going on, consequently becoming lost.

"I can't think right, Mother. Something's wrong with my brain," he said. "I try, but sometimes everything is blurred in my head. I can't concentrate, I just can't. Mother, I want to learn—please help me!" And then he would start to cry.

In these moments, I would put my arm around him and try to bolster his courage. I explained that we all had trouble thinking straight sometimes.

"Don't let it distress you, Billy. You have a *good*

mind, and we'll do our best to help." I tried to reassure *myself* along with him.

The terror of it all was in watching him continuously strain against this restrictive force that leveled each step he tried to climb. I could see the destructive energy within him as plain as day. It would upset him, and as he struggled with its terrible frustrating effect, he would go into temper tantrums horrible to behold and impossible to control.

The habit of incessant erasing, which had begun in the last few months of third grade, persisted into the fourth. While working, he either rubbed holes in his papers or started a lesson over and over again, throwing away his first attempts. Unless it was a report that had to be done perfectly in ink, we urged him to cross out his error and go on from there. But we could not persuade him to do it, and he erased on, compulsively. He *did* seem to know what his homework assignments were, a great improvement over third grade.

Billy also learned to use reference books to supplement subject matter presented in class. He had a set of encyclopedias appropriate for his age, and I had purchased two other sets of reference books he had required. They contained information about all the countries of the world, plus stories of American history and our presidents. He liked to read, and used the books constantly. Generally, if he brought home reading work, I would peruse it first. When he completed his reading, I would ask him questions about its content. I found he usually understood the meaning of the text.

He particularly liked history and geography. One subject we never helped him with was spelling. He had a natural flair for it and did well. Arithmetic, his real skull rattler, was the mean stumbling block.

Bill had spent many hours, slowly—not always

quietly—teaching our son arithmetic, but I could see a change this year in Billy's attitude towards his help. He knew he needed assistance, but at the same time he disliked the necessity for it. He let out many a torrent of words at his dad, his resentment growing every evening he asked for help.

"Now look, Billy, you know your times tables, and division is not any more difficult. Relax, and let's go over that problem again." Bill always began on an optimistic note.

Billy gritted his teeth after the third or fourth time around, broke his pencil in half and ran out of the room. "I don't understand what you mean! I can't do it, I can't! I hate it!" Billy's fustration level was soon reached.

"Come on, Billy, you're not a quitter. Let's have another crack at it," his father encouraged. But then his voice rose in frustration. "Remember, you *asked* me to help."

After a careful explanation of the problem, Billy became very hostile and angry, mostly at himself, for not understanding it right away. This happened almost every night, until I could not bear the agitation they went through. They danced to the same tune endlessly. When Billy got stuck on a problem, he would literally beg his father for help. The explanation over, he was incensed at his failure to understand immediately. This discouraged him to such an extent that he began to loathe the subject. My husband and I argued over this problem until we were at swords' points. There seemed no way out of the arithmetic dilemma.

Most of Billy's teachers were of the opinion that children like our son learned when they were ready. My husband said this was a lot of nonsense. Basically, Billy wanted to learn, or he would not have asked for help.

His father found, as I did, that after the initial frustration was conquered, Billy mastered the basic concepts. Left alone, he floundered and learned nothing. Eventually, real failure would occur. His father was not about to let this happen, in spite of my asking him not to help him so much. He loudly demanded to know how he could get out of it. And I didn't know what to say. Strange as it was, after each arithmetic session and verbal battle, Billy would thank his father for his help and appear happy that he had learned something new.

If he became upset in school, struggling with the same subject, and one of the children tried to assist him, he always refused their help. If his teacher came to his rescue, he graciously accepted.

Usually he worked very slowly in class, and if he had not completed one task before the next was presented, he refused to go on to it. His teacher, knowing his problem, allowed him to stick with whatever he was doing until he finished, whenever it was possible, in order to relieve his unabated torture over his school work.

By fourth grade Billy was so set in his methods of work, he could not change, regardless of what was going on in class. As the work load increased toward the end of the year, his discontent with himself grew. Sometimes he would lie on the floor in class and cry. I assume this happened more than once, although I was unaware of it at the time. Michael's mother told me of Billy's behavior much later. She said his teacher would get so disgusted with his actions at times that she would tell him to take his work and go home. As this information came my way, I pondered again the school psychologist's words, "Leave the teaching to the teachers." Although ours undoubtedly was an exceptional case, I could not understand why they tried to hide from me what was going on in class. I could appreciate the teacher's plight, for more than once I thought one needed the patience of God to reach Billy. But he was *not* hopeless —he *could* learn.

Some of the things he learned that year I wish he hadn't, especially hygiene. It was a new subject for Billy. The study of good personal habits, the existence of germs in our world, the importance of proper food, adequate rest, and general cleanliness were discussed in class. After hygiene was introduced, I noticed Billy washing his hands every twenty minutes while he was at home. He had never liked playing in dirt as a young child, but this was ridiculous.

The more knowledge he acquired, the more bizarre his behavior became. He would go into the bathroom and flush the toilet every ten minutes or so. Every day he asked me if his clothes were clean. He interrogated me incessantly about the cleanliness of his personal articles—toothbrushes, washcloths, towels, etc. He wanted to know if I was absolutely certain that everything was spotless. His obsession carried over into every phase of living. If anyone sneezed, he would leave the room. When he attended church with his father, he walked right out in the middle of the service if he heard someone cough close by. His dad let him go rather than create a scene. When we were eating meals, he refused to touch a crumb if it fell from his plate onto the tabletop. He cringed and backed away if I cleared my throat. If his father, or anyone else, breathed in his direction, he had a fit, and was not above telling strangers or relatives not to get too close.

One evening, as he and his father were working head to head on arithmetic, Billy started to wave his hands back and forth, as one would use a fan.

"What are you doing, Billy?" his father questioned, watching the hands fanning the air.

"I'm chasing germs away," was his answer.

"Come on now, don't be silly," his father said. "I'm breathing the same air you are, and the germs aren't bothering me. What makes you think your germs are special? Now stop that, and let's get to work."

Along with the germ mania came a fear of human contact. He would not hug us—not that he had ever been really affectionate—and heaven forbid that you should kiss him on the cheek! He would be horrified. If it hadn't been so serious, it would have been hilarious. As it was, sometimes we had to turn away from him so that he would not see us laughing.

"Billy, you know mother sees to it that you are properly cared for. Remember all those shots you had to protect your body from illness? That's why the doctor gave them to you—so you would not become ill. Besides, you've already had the measles, mumps and chicken pox, and it's extremely doubtful you'll ever get them again, so why be afraid?" No answer. "Didn't your teacher tell you in class that the human body has a natural immunity to many germs if you are healthy? You know the doctor says you are." Still no answer.

This remained the year of the bugs for us. I could talk myself blue in the face, but Billy remained unconvinced. I began to hate hygiene as much as he hated arithmetic. I had never seen a subject in school have such a debilitating effect on a pupil. He became the worst hypochondriac I have ever known, always afraid that he was about to contract some incurable disease. The dying Camille had nothing on him.

Oh well, life had an occasional better moment. About the middle of the year, Billy's class had to give a performance for the rest of the school. Each child was required to participate. They decided to do *The Mikado,* which meant that all the children had to sing. Billy had a nice voice and carried a tune well, but he was nervous about singing in front of anyone.

"You won't be alone, Billy," I explained. "All the other children have to sing too."

He was unconvinced.

"No, I won't do it! They'll laugh at me." No, no. Negative. Negative. How could I expect anything else? But I kept trying.

"With a nice voice like yours, no one is going to laugh at you, Billy. Of course you can do it. It should be fun, too!" Even as I spoke, I agonized for him.

Had there been a way out, he would have reneged. He couldn't, and this threw him into a tizzy. Anyhow, I made him a blue kimono for his costume, and on the day of the play, I put white powder on his face and black make-up on his eyes. He told me the make-up was necessary. When I took him to school that afternoon, ready for the play, some of the children were not yet made-up or dressed. Billy became upset, thinking he had made a mistake. All the others assured him he was supposed to have his make-up and costume on, but he was so unsure of himself he started to cry and run around in circles of confusion. For a moment I thought he would run right out of the building, but with help, he managed to pull himself together. I left him in the teacher's hands and headed for the auditorium.

To my great surprise and pleasure, Billy sang his part with the group well, never missing a word or note, as he kept time by nodding his head with each beat. When the performance was over, and the audience applauded, he smiled from ear to ear. I never thought I would see the day when Billy could stand still long enough to sing in front of anyone, let alone be happy about it.

That night at supper, I told his father about the show. "He was magnificent, if I do say so myself, Bill. I wish you could have been there." I couldn't help bragging just a little.

"I'm not surprised," he said. And then he turned toward Billy. "Haven't we always told you you could do anything you wanted to? You should trust us, Billy, *and* yourself. We have complete confidence in you." Bill was beaming with pride at his son's accomplishment.

Billy gave me a strong hug and a kiss on the cheek, a singular honor. I could have cried! For a moment our little boy lost had found himself.

It was not all roses, though. In the fourth grade, Billy was not exempt from the teasing he had suffered in past years. Not all the kids teased or ridiculed him, but enough of them did. Some even gave him an encouraging word when he did something right, but that was the exception rather than the rule.

He had been in class with many of the same group for several years, and the children knew his emotional weakness. A few capitalized on it, as those boys had the year before. The fourth grade teacher stood for none of this in class; in fact, she encouraged the children to help Billy, but she couldn't be with them every minute. It was particularly bad on the playground. Sometimes they hounded him until he lost control completely.

One day during the winter, a classmate ripped off Billy's hat and would not return it. Billy chased the boy about, begging for his hat. The more he begged, the more the other child laughed at him, until my son became furious. Seconds later the bell rang, but by then Billy was livid. His tantalizer, satisfied that he had thoroughly upset his victim, tossed the hat back. Billy was wildly angry at the boy, but could not vent his rage in the other child's direction, so he threw his hat on the ground and jumped on it and kicked it, over and over again, shrieking and crying the whole time.

At this point, my aunt appeared and tried to quiet him. It took her a long time. In the meantime, some woman happened along, observing only the last part of the incident. She took one long look at my son, and made some snide comment about his needing a good spanking. My aunt ignored her, as we had all learned to ignore the public's general reaction to Billy's scenes. What a pity they didn't know what they were watching! Perhaps they would not have been so quick to judge him. I had given up explanations long ago, but in order to avoid too much of this sort of thing, I kept Billy home at lunchtime long enough for him to have only sufficient time to lock his bicycle and get into line before the return bell rang. This was avoiding the issue, but it saved him grief and unnecessary torment. Frankly, I did not know what else to do about it.

There were debits this year, but the credit side of our ledger was better than ever before. Billy was still riding his bicycle to school, only now, no one took it away from him. He also learned to lock it and never lost the key. I purchased a house key for him too. Allowing him to unlock the door and enter the house alone might give him a little self-confidence, I thought, but my main purpose was to find out if he would be all right alone. I could never tell when an emergency might arise, and I could not be there to greet him. He had so many fears, and in the past had proved so unreliable at following instructions, that I had to test him. At first I would get in the car and ride around the block to wait a short time beyond the hour he was due home. Then I would return to see if he had gotten in all right. It worked like a charm.

He was much better about bringing home his possessions too. During the first three years of school he had lost enough gloves, hats, boots, and scarves to open a haberdashery. Now, with the exception of a stolen pair of gloves, he did much better. Somehow, too, he had learned the appropriateness of certain things without my telling him. In school he never addressed his aunt by her first name or as "aunty" in front of the others. He always called her "Miss." She had his class for penmanship that year and reported to me many of the things he was doing in school. She said he was always polite to the other children but not friendly toward any except Tommy, Michael, and a new boy, Christopher. For some reason, he liked these three and often asked them to come home to play with him. For the first time since that terrible experience in the next block, he began to ask to go to the other boys' homes to play, too. I was glad of this. His first ventures were in Michael's direction.

At their age, the boys engaged in games of war with helmets, plastic guns, and all. When I called Michael's home one day to tell Billy it was time for supper, Michael's father and I got into a discussion about the boys and how they played. He could not get over how Billy really *lived* the part he took in their war games. Unlike the others, whose interest in such play was superficial and temporary, Billy acted out his extreme emotional torments and fantasies. His anger, which frightened him since he did not know how to handle it, his pent-up frustrations, which he could not express in normal ways, he expressed through the character he assumed in fantasy. He became Hitler, Mussolini, or the Japanese emperor. In this, revenge was his, for he got back at the world he found so painful to live in. His actions represented his concept of the cruelty inflicted upon him by others. This was how the world treated him. He had no other means of coping with his agony, and play was a release for him. In these portrayals he was ruthless, cunning, cruel—the exact opposite of what he truly was. He did not play like this often, but as Michael's father said, it was amazing to watch. He was Doctor Jekyll and Mr. Hyde, two distinct personalities.

I had observed this myself when Christopher, Michael, Tommy, and Billy got together. Usually they had a great time, but Billy was always isolated, emotionally speaking. He had just about every game or toy that would make most children happy, but he seldom showed interest in them—a carry-over from when he was little. When the boys came to play, they used his toys. He would stick with them for a while, but usually wandered off to play by himself with his science kit or to paint pictures, using the oil colors he had received the previous Christmas. He never seemed to resent their using his things, and he certainly enjoyed their presence.

Watching the four of them was a real study in character development. Christopher was Billy's type, shy. Tommy and Michael were aggressive. But they all accepted Billy's ways without question. If Billy was displeased or upset, they could quiet him down faster than I could. Christopher and Billy were becoming fast friends when, to our great disappointment, Chris moved to another state.

One day Billy told me how much he had liked Christopher, and how he missed him. In all the years I had been watching Billy grow, I could not remember his expressing such affection for another person. I was touched by his loneliness.

Billy was now 10 years old. Up to this time, we had not asked him to take the responsibility for any household chores. We felt he had all he could do to manage his school work, but the time had come to trust him with small tasks. I began to send him to the store on his bicycle for one or two items, such as bread or milk. I wanted him to learn how to buy things and get the proper change. Besides, I thought it might help him with his arithmetic. We also asked him to take out the refuse and dry the dishes—not every night, but when he had the time. In return, he received a small allowance. When he had saved enough money, he went to the store with his father or me, and bought a plastic model kit.

A few times, I watched him assemble a car, ship, or plane replica with a deftness that was wonderful to behold. He would read the instructions, carefully glue the parts together, sometimes using tweezers as he worked, and then paint the finished product. Some of these structures had many oddly shaped pieces. It was engrossing to watch him busily at work. One ship, a brigantine, turned out to be a masterpiece. I had never seen him work so carefully before. After he glued all the parts together, he took his tweezers and black string to tie the sails, placing string wherever rope was used on this type of vessel. He did a beautiful job and kept this model for many years.

"That's perfect, Billy," I praised him.

"I know, Mom. I think I'll put it on my bookcase," he replied, proud of his achievement.

Billy's interest in model building was replacing his pencil drawing as a spare time occupation. It was a creative outlet for him, a means of telling others he was capable. His pal, Tommy, marvelled at the neatness of his work, and, frankly, so did I. When I thought about the innumerable school papers with holes in them from excessive erasing, I was stumped by the concentration and skill he showed putting models together. However, in Billy's case, one area of endeavor never carried over to another. Each was a thing apart. His personality was the same—a hodgepodge of shattered pieces. No amount of effort on his part or ours could restore the pieces to a complete composite.

When Billy discovered models, he also discovered the movies. Occasionally his father or I would take Tom and Billy downtown on a Saturday afternoon so they could see a show. When the movie was over, we returned to pick them up. We carefully screened the type of pictures we allowed him to see, because we did not want him to get upset.

One particular Saturday, Billy wanted to go to a Walt Disney picture, but Tommy could not go with him. I knew the movie had a sad ending, and was reluctant to let him go alone.

"What's the matter with you? You encourage him to step out on his own, and now you think he shouldn't see a simple movie?" Bill and I were at it again.

"It's not that, Bill, but the picture has a sad ending, and I don't think he should see it. You know how he is." I didn't want to argue, but—

"I say he goes." With that, his father overruled me.

When his dad went to pick him up after the movie, Billy got into the car without saying a word. Suddenly, he burst out crying, so angry with us for letting him go that he raged on for hours.

The picture upset him so deeply he could not tolerate it. We tried to explain that movies were only stories, not necessarily real or true, but he did not understand. He only knew that he could not watch misery and sorrow taking place on the screen, for he knew from firsthand experience what it meant to feel pain. It took two days for us to get him to see reason. I was angry with myself for giving in to his father. I should have known better. For years afterward, Billy refused to go to the movies at all.

Many, many times my husband and I disagreed on

methods of handling our son. It occurred to me that we talked about, and fought about, practically nothing else. We did make a concerted effort not to argue in front of Billy. It was difficult, sometimes impossible, to remain silent in his presence, especially if there was a clash of wills or opinions. In our infinite concern for his well-being, we lashed at one another, both of us feeling helpless when we could not penetrate Billy's torment.

My husband's personality was more forceful than my own, but on one issue I bulldozed my will over his. During 1964 the necessity for orthodontia for Billy became a prime source of dissension between us. We had a continual terrific verbal battle about it. Billy was a handsome child, but his front teeth protruded, and he was having difficulty pronouncing certain letters of the alphabet. His speech patterns were stilted anyhow, but as I corrected him, and he tried to correct himself, I could see that the problem was due to the placement of his teeth. He could not pronounce "th" and used the letter "f" as a substitute. He had similar trouble with "b" and "v." As I pushed the discussions on this subject, my husband's temper flared.

"No! Absolutely no! He has enough problems already." Bill was almost shouting at me. "What in the name of God do you think it will be *like,* trying to get him through *that* ordeal? I won't hear of it! Three years of going to the dentist? Are you out of your mind? Don't we have enough to handle now?" He adamantly refused to have Billy's teeth straightened. But I could be just as stubborn as he.

"I don't give a damn what you say! It has to be done! He's having trouble talking already, and if we let him go, he'll look like Bugs Bunny for the rest of his life! I say *it will be done,* and you can go to the devil! I'll pay for it myself." It would have been hard to find any love between us as the argument continued.

"Listen, it's not the money," Bill pleaded. "I tell you *he'll never make it,* and he's a little better, so why do you insist on making him miserable?" Was he accusing me of wanting something *not* in Billy's best interest? I was more determined than ever.

"I am his mother, and I say it is going to be done! We've gotten him this far; we can get him through this." That was all I had to say.

"I'm warning you, Jessie, you'd better not start anything you can't finish." It sounded like a threat, but at least the argument had terminated. I had had a part time job working in a laboratory at night ever since Billy was five years old. It had been my salvation in many a bad year, an excuse to get away from household confusion, and to collect my jangled nerves and thoughts. I was, therefore, ready, willing, and able to take care of this matter myself, with or without my husband's approval.

It took three years to complete the teeth-straightening operation. One real crisis arose when the orthodontist told me my son would have to have four teeth removed before the work could proceed further. I did not know how Billy or his father would take this news.

My husband had a fit, of course, but he didn't worry me. I had made up my mind to go through with it. But I wondered how we could get Billy through another surgical ordeal with only minimal difficulty.

The orthodontist recommended a dental surgeon, and Billy's father took him for the first appointment early in May, 1965. My husband explained our son's emotional problems to the surgeon in case he did not wish to handle him. Billy was a challenge, the doctor admitted, but he was ready to meet it. While they were discussing what anesthetic to use, Billy piped up and said he wanted novocaine, because his regular dentist used it, and he was not afraid of that.

The removal of the upper and lower bicuspids with novocaine was an impractical procedure, so the dentist told my husband to bring Billy prepared for a general anesthetic, and he would see how things went. I took Billy to the surgeon's office on May 7th. When we entered, the nurse took him into the inner office. As usual, my heart was in my throat, waiting to hear Billy start screaming. Time passed, and I heard absolutely nothing. The silence was deafening, and my anxiety grew to unbearable proportions as I waited. Ages passed before the nurse reappeared and asked me to come in. She said Billy had really put himself to sleep and never mentioned novocaine even once. Would wonders never cease?

The surgeon had done an excellent job. Billy's mouth did not bleed afterward, nor did he complain of excessive pain. My husband could not believe it had all gone so smoothly. After this surgery, the rest was easy.

The next three years of dental visits passed quickly. Billy wanted his teeth to look right and never expressed annoyance with the metal braces and rubber bands or other paraphernalia that made his mouth look like an overstocked hardware store. He was conscientious about cleaning his teeth, and, in this instance, his hypochondria worked in his favor. I have always been glad I held out to have his teeth straightened, and in recent years, he has thanked me for my insistence. That was one of several arguments worth winning.

7

All the Wrong Decisions

Every week of 1964 and part of 1965, we three spent an hour with our son's psychiatrist. The doctor felt Billy was old enough to hear what we had to say about him and to contribute his own thoughts and feelings to our discussions. Shall we call it group therapy? It was our contention, and the doctor's, that by working openly together, we might be able to alleviate the boy's countless fears and to redirect his confused and inappropriate thought processes. Theoretically, it sounded plausible, very promising, but in practice it was not a successful venture. We talked, argued, and debated, but Billy changed little, and after a year the tide began to turn. It seemed to my husband and to me that we were progressing backward. In all honesty, I don't think his psychiatrist agreed with us, but *we* lived with Billy, *he* did not. Billy's behavior improved for a while, and then he retrogressed again.

Among the improvements that gave us a little peace was the cessation of his awful nightmares. He even gained enough courage to sleep in his own bed. His relationships and communicative powers with others did not improve, nor did he stop being under unending stress of one sort or another in school.

We would praise him constantly, and he would make

a little surge forward, but then he would withdraw into a safe, dependent relationship again. The step ahead was lost as he retreated for protection—against what, we did not know. Our experiences with Billy in 1964 were the best so far, but his uncertainty about himself and his world remained constant. All of us working together could not push him in the right direction. He was growing *older*, not really growing *up*. He was a challenge to all of us, including his psychiatrist.

As a result of 1964's group therapy, Billy began to talk openly about his problems. This was both good and bad. He talked incessantly, wildly, compulsively, with frequent repetition, until he nearly drove us mad. He followed me around the house, chattering like a magpie, interrupting me on the telephone, any time, any place. He would tell stories concerning some fantasy that troubled him, or just complain about things in general. He paused only for eating, sleeping, and taking care of necessities. *He* never tired, but we did. When he was especially wound up, he followed us to bed, uninvited, and continued to talk even after the lights were out. He talked and paced until we insisted that he go to bed. Sometimes his father had to move him forcibly to his own room and bed.

If he started a story one night, he awoke the next morning and began where he had left off. If and when he finally finished, he would interrogate us to see if we had been listening carefully. If we goofed on an answer —one needed a mind like a steel trap to hold all he said —he became angry, extremely perturbed, often going into a temper tantrum. No one will ever know how I wished to flee from the sound of his voice! Had I been able to fool him, I would have resorted to stuffing my ears with cotton, blocking out the noise; but there was no escape. His father, bless him, had greater tolerance and fortitude, listening to Billy for hours on end.

This nonstop verbal rambling had a strange quality about it. His stories were expressed in stylized narrative form, and for years, if someone asked him a question or spoke to him, he responded in a long, involved manner, including facts not pertinent to the original question or comment. Occasionally his answer had nothing to do with the question at all. It drove me wild when he could not get to a conclusion or make his point without taking the long way around. I tried my best to hold my impatience in check and not to express annoyance. Being human, I didn't find it easy. On the other hand, there were some days when he would not talk at all.

When Billy went out with me, and we met a friend, he would start discussing his troubled state and thoughts. I had to tell him we didn't do this. "Billy, dear, we mustn't talk outside of our home about these feelings you have. Other people have their problems too, and they are not really interested in ours."

It was hard to get this across. In his mind, it seemed the right thing to do. After all, when we went to the psychiatrist he was encouraged, urged, to talk. Why not now? A full confession of his miseries was forced upon every available ear. I had a problem explaining his odd communications to the verbally assaulted victim.

Strangely enough Billy did not do much talking at school. His teacher had trouble extracting responses from him. She *did* comment that his deportment was better, and he no longer stuck out like a sore thumb from the others.

The end of fourth grade marked the turning point in Billy's schooling, because of two factors. Before the close of school, all pupils were required to take achievement tests. Under tension while taking the examinations, Billy was unusually distractible. We were cautioned not to expect much in the way of scores. His teacher felt they would not reflect the real progress he had made during the year. His report card had been excellent, but his father and I knew the exertion, the hours of dedication, it had taken to keep him up scholastically. We felt he was bright, surprisingly so, considering all things; but reaching him, getting him to produce, was pure bedlam.

The second factor involved the rearrangement of the whole local school system to obtain racial balance. Ordinarily, our son would have attended his neighborhood school through the sixth grade, but integration intervened. Billy would be transferred for fifth and sixth grade to another school nearly a mile away, and transferred also for junior and senior high school. We were deeply concerned.

"I know you could drive him to school, Jessie, but sometimes he might have to walk. I don't like the idea; it's too far. Every time he goes more than a couple of blocks away, he gets into some kind of a mess," my husband began.

"I don't like it either, Bill, but what can we do about it?" I asked. "They're going to change the whole school system around, and it's that school or none." I was already reconciled to the inevitable.

"Jessie, it's not just the long walk," Bill protested. "We just can't keep on helping him so much with his school work. He's never going to make it! I know him, and, as sure as I'm sitting here, he'll be in trouble in two weeks! I'm going to ask his psychiatrist to get the scores on his achievement tests and then we're going to have to make some sort of a decision about this!"

Was I hearing correctly? Had Bill given up on his son?

"You know, sometimes I don't understand you," I told him. "You're the one who's always telling me I don't have enough faith in him. And all of a sudden, you won't give him a chance to try a new school. Why?" I couldn't understand, but I shrugged my shoulders and acquiesced. "I think you're jumping the gun—Billy really did better this year; but let's get the test results and see how bad things really are!"

We had a private conference with Billy's doctor to air the matter. He based his judgment of our son's progress on his report cards in spite of our protestations that they presented an inaccurate picture. I assume he felt we overexaggerated our son's inadequacies. He said we would have another meeting when he received the test scores. Meanwhile, he suggested that we give Billy a chance to prove his ability to go it alone by sending him to summer camp. It sounded like a good idea.

We looked around at several before deciding on the Y.M.C.A. camp in New York State. It was well run, and Billy had never had any difficulties while attending activities at the local Y.M.C.A. We made arrangements, with Billy's approval, to send him for two weeks in July. I talked to Billy about what fun was in store for him, trying to stir his enthusiasm. I was also trying to control my own anxiety about sending him away for the first time. If he *did* make it alone, it would be a tremendous step forward. I had my doubts; my husband didn't. We were always altering positions that way.

We drove the two hundred miles or so to camp and took Billy to the indoctrination building. There the camp nurse checked each child, taking his temperature, and recording any special medical instructions to be followed. On our application we had stated Billy's problem so the staff would know what to do with him if an emergency occurred. We included the name, address, and phone number of his psychiatrist.

While waiting to be processed, Billy met another boy from our hometown. He seemed happy to see a familiar face. I was pleased too, knowing he would not feel completely strange and alone. I could see him relax as he began to talk to the other boy.

Before starting on the trip, we had made reservations to stay close by the first night. My husband thought I was ridiculous, but I wanted to make sure Billy survived the first night before I could relax. The sounds of happy children shouting and singing at the lodge eased my tension. It was a camp rule that children were not allowed to call their parents for any reason. Only if the camp director felt it was an absolute necessity would they get in touch with the parents.

The next two weeks passed slowly for me. The house was so quiet I could not wait for Billy to return. I had often thought what heaven it would be to lead a quiet, normal life. I was surprised to find myself missing Billy, wandering about in the empty silence, wondering what to do with my free moments.

My husband experienced the same sensation. It had never dawned on us before how much time we devoted to Billy, ignoring each other's needs in our mutual relentless desire to help him.

As the days dragged along, I wondered why we had not received a note from him. The children were encouraged to write home. When one week had passed, we received a letter from his counselor, who said Billy was doing fine. The news was better than I had expected, but I still felt uneasy.

His father and grandfather drove to camp and picked him up when his two weeks were over. Billy was relatively silent on the long ride home. About two blocks from our house he broke into tears, and as they pulled into the driveway, I heard him screaming.

He ran into the house, and I nearly collapsed as he passed me. He must have lost twenty pounds! He was skin and bones, little more, and covered with the marks of insect bites. His clothes were filthy, but I had anticipated that.

"Why did you send me to that stupid camp? I hated it! I hate it! I hate you!" His tirade went on and on.

That night he woke up shrieking hideously. I thought his nightmares were returning, so I called his psychiatrist the next morning.

"He's experiencing a perfectly natural trauma. It happens to lots of kids the first time they're away from home. It'll pass in a few days. At least we know he managed to survive," he said.

The crying and raging lasted five weeks. Billy thought, in his twisted way, that we had wanted to punish him. He felt we didn't love him, in spite of the encouraging letters we had written to him. Hours of explanations, and praise for sticking it out, were necessary before he forgave us.

When the camp season was over, I called his counselor to find out what had happened. He couldn't understand it himself. The first week Billy was the best kid he had. He did everything he was asked to do and was very cooperative. The second week he seemed to fall apart, crying and wandering around like a lost, homesick soul.

"That's what we get for listening to others—" I told my husband, "a miserable kid and weeks of sleepless nights." He just looked at me, disgusted.

To get Billy's mind off his troubles, we spent the rest of the summer taking him places we thought he would enjoy. The World's Fair was first on our list. It was great! Billy was interested in everything, especially the Disneyland dinosaurs in the Ford Building.

"What makes them move, Pop? How do they build them to look so real? Can they really walk, or do they just stand there and move?" The questions went on and on.

One Disney exhibit, "It's a Small World" turned into a calamity for Billy. In a way, it was my fault. To see "It's a Small World," we rode in a boat through a building where there were doll-like puppets dancing and singing, representing people from all over the world. The music was very loud, and before I realized what was happening, Billy grabbed his ears and doubled over screaming, with his head down between his knees. He continued to scream during the rest of the ride. When we emerged, he was beside himself with distress, and ran down the walk away from the building as fast as he could. We chased after him. Until that moment I had forgotten how he had reacted to the noon whistle years before. It took us more than an hour to calm him down. Finally he got over being upset and rode on a few of the amusements with us. With that one exception, however, he enjoyed everything. He snapped out of the depression into which camp had pushed him. At home, he resumed playing with his pal Tom. Together, they always thought of something to do.

One Saturday afternoon they asked us if they could rent a tandem and ride in the park about four blocks from our home. I did not trust some types of characters to be found in the park, but my husband scoffed, "What can happen to them in broad daylight?"

I felt I should not deny my son's wishes just to pacify my own fears so I agreed to let them go. They had been gone about half an hour when I heard Billy hollering. This time Tommy was yelling too. They came up the driveway full speed, as if the devil himself was chasing them.

While they had been riding in the park, some older boys had stopped them. They had threatened to burn Billy with their cigarettes if he and Tom did not give up the tandem. They took the bicycle from the boys, and when they were finished with it, threw it into the lake. Luckily, another big fellow, one who knew Billy and Tommy, came along. He chased the bullies off, but not before the bike had been dunked.

What can happen in broad daylight indeed! That did it for me. From then on we did not allow the boys to ride alone. Someone older had to go with them if they left our block. Billy seemed to be a magnet for trouble.

As summer drew to a close, we had to start thinking about the next school year. The rearrangement of the school system created pressing problems. But our main concern was Billy's immaturity and his dependence on us for academic support. We were willing and able to help, but both of us feared our assistance wasn't helping Billy grow up.

We welcomed our next conference with Billy's psychiatrist. This time he had the scores of Billy's tests. He was quite surprised at the test results, but we were not. Billy scored in the lower ten per cent of his class. It was obvious to us that the discrepancy between his report cards and these scores was due to our constantly helping him. What he had needed, for a long time, was schooling designed for the emotionally disturbed. But nothing of this type existed where we lived.

Billy's psychiatrist recommended immediate placement in a residential school or a day school that handled children with problems like his. I was hesitant to agree, remembering my husband's earlier comment,

"What are you getting so upset about? He's the same boy we've always had."

We *had* struggled along with him so far. Couldn't we allow him to continue in public school as long as he didn't completely fall apart? His father said, "Absolutely not!" His psychiatrist agreed! They seemed in league against me.

I was dead set against a residential school. I was afraid to release my son to someone else's indifferent care. I told the psychiatrist and my husband that I would consider a day school, however. The doctor felt that Billy's camp experience proved that he could handle a residential situation. I felt it proved exactly the opposite. Again, my husband agreed with the psychiatrist. But I won the argument.

After this conference, and before making our final decision, we asked our board of education if there was any special training available for Billy locally. They said there was not. We began to search for the best day school for our son and settled on one in South Orange, New Jersey.

I took Billy for an interview, and, after testing, he was accepted for the following year. We had to sign a contract agreeing to pay $1,500.00. If he was withdrawn for any reason, we would still be required to pay the full amount. Before signing, we had a long talk with the school's directress. We explained Billy's needs for individual instruction, and the difficulties he had trying to function in a large group. I had her call Billy's psychiatrist to get a complete picture of our child before agreeing to work with him. I told her it was our wish to leave the teaching to the teachers.

She assured us that each student began instruction on his own level of achievement in each subject, and was brought up to grade from that point. The work was done in small groups, allowing ample time for individual instruction. Homework was a rarity. If a concept was not understood, it was repeated until the child grasped it. The approach sounded like an answer to our prayers.

Even after we had signed the contract, Billy's psychiatrist continued to pressure us to consider a residential school. I stubbornly refused. I felt our son was too immature and insecure to be torn away from his home—the only safety he had felt. Billy's psychiatrist insisted that a change of environment would awaken the child and help him become independent. I did not agree. He considered Billy a borderline compensated schizophrenic, which meant that he could function in normal society in a limited way. He warned that Billy tottered on a wire. One misstep could throw him into a hopeless state. Proceeding on this premise, I thought that wrenching the boy from his home and family could be catastrophic for him. In the end, the psychiatrist yielded. We could forestall residential school as long as Billy continued to function at a reasonable level.

Billy was crushed and bewildered when we told him he would be going to private school. "I don't want to go to some old dumb school! I want to go with my friends and Tommy," he protested.

"Listen, Billy," his father explained. "You know your mother and I want you to be happy, and you know how you don't like having us help you with school work. Wouldn't you rather go to a school where you can get some help from your teachers?"

"I guess so—but who's going to take me anyhow?" With that final reluctance he accepted our decision.

It really seemed promising, but there was a hitch— I would be driving sixty miles a day to take Billy to school and bring him home—three hundred miles a

week. I was willing, but as time passed, it became difficult to keep up the pace.

Billy did not particularly like the new school. When
the homework began to pile up, I could see his anger
and disgust mounting. We were once again drawn into
the whirlpool. It was developing into the old rat race,
and it seemed to us that the school's policies had been
falsely stated. When I confronted the school's directress
on the point of homework, she asked me, "Why can't
you just sit quietly by his side, and encourage him as he
works?" I could have screamed!

Before settling on the South Orange school, we had
tried, without success, to find a nearby program of education for emotionally disturbed children. We wondered
why no attempts were being made to provide facilities
for them within the local school system.

"What do other people *do* who have problems like
this?" my husband asked. "I'm sure there are many
more like Billy."

"I don't know," I confessed, "but we're lucky we
have the financial resources to help him—if you can call
it help. I don't know, Bill, I'm really getting discouraged
with this learning business—they tell us one thing and
do another." It was *so* frustrating to me. "I should think
it would be more sensible if they helped troubled kids
when they're young, in their own community, instead of
waiting until the problems are out of hand and the kids
become dropouts. I wonder, like you do, what happens
to other kids like ours."

Bill shrugged at the hopelessness of it. "They are
shunted aside, I guess, and ignored. If they're not lucky,
they eventually end up in a prison or become the responsibility of society." How could a society do this to
its children?

Some of the questions that bounced around in my head were about to be answered for me.

September was gone, and as October began, my health began to deteriorate. The strain of driving three hundred miles a week plus tending to household duties, working nights, looking after my father-in-law, and worrying about Billy was taking its toll. My doctor became concerned that I would literally fall apart. I felt that way myself.

In September my husband had written to the Deputy Commissioner of Education for the State of New Jersey, requesting busing aid for our handicapped child. We had hoped to obtain transportation help under the Beadleston Act and the Grossi Amendment, but, unfortunately, emotionally disturbed children were not covered by their provisions. The following year, 1966, a new law did include busing and education programs for emotionally disturbed and socially maladjusted children. At the present there is still a large gap between the intent and the application of the legislation, but with time, it will work. When we were struggling, there was nothing.

As the days wore on, and I wore down, my husband once again went to the local board to ask for help with getting Billy to school. Our request for assistance was turned down, but as a result of our inquiry we received a letter from the school board's psychiatric social worker. She stated that they might have a beneficial educational plan for Billy and asked us to meet with her to discuss it.

We learned that while we had been looking for a school for our son, our home town was making plans to start a class for emotionally disturbed youngsters. Now that I could no longer keep up with getting Billy to school, they offered us a place for him in this special class. They had obtained a teacher, specially trained and qualified to handle children with special problems.

The class would have four students at the beginning —two aggressive and two withdrawn personality types, our son fitting the latter category. Later, the number would be raised to eight, the legal limit for such classes. They proposed that having opposing personality types within the group would benefit each child's character development. In theory, the constant interaction of varying emotional behavior would contribute to the improved deportment and development of each student. The very small number of pupils allowed the teacher adequate time to give individual help. As the year passed, they intended to reintegrate these children into a regular class, for a small part of each day at first, ultimately returning them full time, depending on the progress each one made.

As the psychiatric social worker talked, I had that "here-we-go-again feeling." I was beginning to mistrust all the proposed "ideal situations" for our son. Inside, I knew Billy was an unbending, unchanging young boy, and I was not impressed with the rather experimental hypothesis on which the class was based. Billy had been playing with very aggressive children for years, and it had not influenced his behavior. Perversely, the more they pushed him, the more he withdrew from them and the realities of life about him. I expressed my objection, but the social worker implored us to give the proposal our fullest consideration. A rejection on our part would be final, and the opportunity would be unavailable to us later because of our son's age. It was now or never. As far as I was concerned, it could be never; my husband felt otherwise.

We were reluctant to start such a program unless it would have dependable continuity. We did not wish to start our son and have him dropped or pushed from one place to another. We requested an interview with the new teacher before making any decision.

The teacher was young and filled with professed dedication and a genuine interest in children, especially disturbed children. What she lacked in experience, she made up for in zeal.

"It is my intention to stay with this work and this school system for many years," she said.

As she talked to us, I kept thinking, "My dear, there is a vast difference between talking a good job and doing it." I was unhappy with the whole idea and skeptical about the results it might produce. My husband's concern for my health overruled my objections, and he enrolled Billy in the class.

When I informed the directress of the South Orange school of my husband's decision, she was horrified. She suggested a riding pool might help me, but I had already called every mother who was driving from my area. They had established pools and did not wish to change their schedules. Accepting this, she was quick to remind me that we had signed a contract, and were legally responsible for the tuition fee. It irked me somewhat to know that the local board could have saved us a considerable amount of money had they informed us of this special class before the school year began.

Billy started to attend the new class at the end of October, 1965. He was happy not to be going to "that cranky old place" anymore. With the change in schools came a change in the psychiatric sessions. Billy now went alone. I guess the psychiatrist had given up on us, but he felt he could still do something for our son. We had told him about the new class, and set up an appointment for the new teacher to see him. A thorough background on our son's illness would help her to understand him.

The first morning, he was taken to school by a driver. He looked scared to death, the original lost soul, as he climbed into the car and waved goodbye. The days went smoothly until an extremely aggressive boy was introduced into the group. He singled Billy out as his personal target, and from then on our son had no peace. His work suffered, and he could ill afford it. As the days passed, he withdrew from class participation of any kind. His tormentor plagued him until he grew listless, uncommunicative, and disinterested in general. He was punched, pinched, and annoyed at every opportunity. He was called "stupid," "retarded," and "dumb" by this tease. What infuriated us was that the teacher allowed this to go on without interruption. I went to school to talk to her about Billy's deteriorating condition. I was alarmed at the outlook Billy was expressing about school at home.

"May I ask you why something isn't done to stop this?" I asked. "I know the atmosphere of a class of this type has to be permissive, but incessant harassment is not helping my son or the other boy, I'm sure." I began as politely as I knew how.

"Mrs. Foy," she replied, her voice carefully controlled, "we are waiting patiently for Billy to defend himself. He must learn to get along with others and defend his rights. If we do it for him, he will never learn."

Apparently, the idea was to back him into a corner, forcing him to come out fighting. Knowing how Billy abhorred and feared violence, I knew they would have a long wait. But my protestations were ignored!

Since we had already withdrawn Billy from South Orange, we could not return him. We were caught again, like rats in a trap. Then his teacher dropped another bomb.

"Really, Mrs. Foy, I think Billy has more than one problem," she offered.

"What do you mean?" I asked.

"I think he has the problem of retardation as well as his emotional disorder," she stated, matter-of-factly.

I exploded. "I don't know *how* you can *make* such an assumption!" I stormed. "I would appreciate it if we could discuss this further, *with* my husband and the principal!"

The one thing we would not tolerate was to have Billy handled as a retarded child. His problems were serious, but he was *not* retarded. How could the teacher think otherwise—especially since she had been fully informed of Billy's condition by his psychiatrist?

In the principal's office, the teacher was informed that her assumptions were incorrect. It was her job to modify Billy's behavior, if possible, not to draw false and unwarranted conclusions. Unconvinced, she agreed to try to help him further. *Right out of his mind,* I thought. I was surprised at my own antagonism toward her.

My son's adversary soon learned about Billy's hypochondria. At every opportunity he blew his breath in Billy's face, or spat at him. Even after our talk, the teacher did nothing to stop it.

How I longed for Billy to fight back! "Billy, I don't care if you think it is not nice or not! You've *got* to hit him back! Right in the face—or he'll *never* leave you alone!" But talking was useless.

"I'm afraid, mother." Billy told me what I already knew. "If I hit him, I'll kill him! I've tried to be his friend, but he only laughs at me and says he doesn't want me to."

"All the more reason you must defend yourself!" I insisted. Our conversation went on and on, getting nowhere.

Instead of seeking retaliation, Billy turned his complete anger on himself, as he had always done. He would come into the house after school and pound his head and chest with his fists, tearing his hair in agony, screaming his frustration. The torment was unbearable. I was beside myself watching him. No wonder Billy gave up! This experiment they were conducting with human nature was flirting with disaster. It was a monstrous miscalculation on their part, not only in my son's case, but for the others as well.

We were enraged that the Child Study Team, directing this program under the supervision of the Assistant Superintendent of Schools, did nothing to correct the situation. Our strenuous objections were dismissed without consideration. How we regretted the move we had made that subjected our child to such treatment! He would carry the scars of emotional carnage with him for years. All the progress Billy had made in the fourth grade disappeared. The slight maturing we had nurtured died. All was lost.

The crowning arrogance was perpetrated upon us in June when his teacher told us that Billy should be back in concentrated therapy. No wonder, after the year he had spent with her! He would not be put back in a regular class. And our son told us flatly that he would never return to school again if he had to spend one minute with that boy. We were sick.

8

The Moment of Truth

Billy's standard operating procedure consisted of heading in a chosen direction, and then turning away from it. He did this so often that it made my head spin to keep up with him. In a way, he did it again during this summer. He asked if he could go back to the Y.M.C.A. camp, after he had sworn he would never return.

We had planned a trip to California during August, but we felt that since Billy expressed the desire to return to camp, we should allow him to do so. Of course he had to have a camp physical. Billy was eleven and a half now, and we decided to change doctors. The new man was very thorough, taking nothing for granted, including what I told him. It was he who discovered my son's myopia. He agreed that the measles had undoubtedly done the damage. I was stunned when I thought of the times Billy had been examined, his defective vision going unnoticed. When he put on his glasses for the first time, he couldn't believe how different everything looked. In spite of corrective lenses, Billy continued to walk in a peculiar fashion part of the time, and shied away from playing ball or having things thrown in his direction. Sometimes he told me objects moved oddly, too, as he looked at them. He wondered why this happened.

As the physician was examining our son, he mentioned two other points he was concerned about. He thought Billy might have slight brain damage. I suggested he get in touch with Billy's psychiatrist to discuss his feelings with him. He also told me my son's blood pressure was extraordinarily high. I remembered that Billy had said to his psychiatrist several times he felt there was something wrong with his heart. We had all dismissed his complaint as another hypochondriac symptom. But this doctor wanted Billy to have a chest X-ray. I was not surprised that Billy had high blood pressure, but the figures the doctor quoted me were alarming. I considered Billy's hyperactivity and being upset ninety per cent of the time enough to drive anyone's blood pressure up. But I was wrong. There was more to it, as I found out years later.

The doctor and the psychiatrist decided it would be wise for Billy to have another neurological examination, including an encephalogram. We postponed the examination until after Billy's camping trip and our trip to California.

Once more we drove him to camp. This time we returned home the same day, leaving him lodged in cabin 13, a step higher up the mountain, with a new counselor. We thought it might be a good experience for him to ride home on the bus with other boys and counselors. I took time to prepare a number of postcards, already addressed to us at home. There was a card for each day— not that I expected him to write that often but so he could let us know how he was getting along, if he wanted to.

A week and a half passed, and we received no card. I was tempted to call the camp.

"No, you are not going to call, and that's that," Bill insisted. "If anything was wrong, they would let us

know. Besides, you'll destroy his confidence if he thinks
we're checking up on him. Now stop the damn fret-
ting!" he scolded me. But confidence was an empty
word when it applied to Billy, and my apprehension
mounted, in spite of Bill's assurances.

I missed the child, as I had the year before, but this
time we were busy visiting schools while he was away.
We were looking for the impossible—a school to both
educate and help him. We did not want to put him back
in that awful class, although he would have a different
"special, trained teacher," and would be in a different
classroom. Most important of all, he would be separated from his archenemy.

We went everywhere, talking ourselves hoarse, without results. Most of the schools were already filled and
had waiting lists. Others did not handle schizophrenic
children. We finally conceded defeat. Having no alternative, we decided to try the program he had been involved in, for one more year.

Our searching over, we sat waiting for the homecom-
ing bus to arrive. I was very much on edge. When it
pulled in, and Billy emerged, I relaxed a bit. He was not
skin and bones, but he had brought the mountain dirt
with him. He didn't cry, and he told us the best part of
the whole two weeks was the bus ride home. Everyone
had given him candy or something to eat. I thought he
had enjoyed himself, but on the short drive home from
the bus station, he said, "I'll never go back to that
dumb, stupid camp again." He had been upset a good
part of the time. He had gotten lost in the woods at
night, going from the mess hall back to his cabin, and
had wandered around in the dark a long while before
getting his bearings.

"Billy, why didn't you send us a post card if you were

so unhappy?" I asked him. "I fixed them so you wouldn't have to bother about getting stamps."

No answer! He would never answer if he did not wish to pursue the subject further. I unpacked his dirt-filled trunk and found the answer myself. On each one of the unmailed post cards he had written how miserable he was. He was afraid he would kill us for letting him go back to camp. Confusing as it may sound, he expressed a great fear that something would happen to us while he was gone. I showed the cards to his father. Both of us were puzzled, because the child had begged to go. Maybe the request was made to prove to himself, or to us, that he could make it alone. I don't know. At least he didn't have nightmares afterwards. He had written out his feelings of hatred, anger, and fear for us and for himself. In that way, he got it out of his sytem. We praised him repeatedly for sticking with it, even while he had been completely unhappy.

I was beginning to speculate on the wisdom of our forthcoming airplane flight. I kept my fingers crossed as I told Billy about all the interesting and wonderful places we would be seeing. We had to prepare him ahead of time for any new experience. Flying would be a new one for him.

We had no problem getting him on the plane; but as the stewardess gave her cheerful talk about needing extra oxygen if we flew too high and explained how the oxygen masks would fall down from the ceiling, Billy was shaken with fear. It was a good thing the engines started about that time. I strapped Billy into his seat, and buried his head in my chest. He could not look as we took off, and he was hollering the whole time. We had flown halfway across the United States before he relaxed enough to look out of the windows. Every once in a while his eyes glanced up at the ceiling. When we landed and disembarked he swore he would never get back on another plane.

My mother was at the airport to greet us. My parents had been divorced when I was ten years old, but over the years we kept in close touch by writing. I had told her all about my son, so she knew what to expect. When they got to know each other, Billy told me he adored his grandmother, especially her soft melodic voice. She had been born in Scotland, and the trace of her homeland had stayed in her soft Scottish accent. They became great friends, although she had some difficulty understanding his wide mood swings and why he acted "different" at times for no apparent reason. It was that "no apparent reason" that always troubled me.

We took Billy all over California, from San Francisco to Long Beach, with a side trip to Catalina Island. We saw Marineland of the Pacific where he fell in love with Bubbles, a huge whale, and Flipper, the dolphin.

"Say, Mom, is that the same Flipper I watch on television?" he wanted to know.

"They say it is, Billy, but they probably use more than one to make the films," I explained.

We toured the movie studios and visited the set where the Munsters, a comic horror show, was made. Strapped to a table was a large replica of Herman Munster. If you pushed a button, the table began to rise. I thought Billy would faint with fright as he watched this taking place. I must admit it was rather macabre to look at. He couldn't get out of there fast enough, even though he had been unafraid of the dummy before it started to move.

When we had covered Los Angeles, where my mother lived, we thought we should head elsewhere. Before exploring further, my mother suggested that we might like to go to Forrest Lawn Cemetery to see the world's largest painting of the crucifixion and another of the resurrection. At first I thought she wasn't serious, but she insisted. *Who wants to visit a cemetery, on a vacation?* I wondered. But it turned out to be the most moving experience imaginable, for more than one reason.

Within the cemetery grounds there is a building containing a large auditorium with a huge stage. As we sat down to wait for the unveiling of the renowned work of art, I began to wonder what I was doing there. After a brief pause, the curtains rolled back slowly, and the lights of the auditorium dimmed. On the stage before us was the largest painting I had ever seen. It covered the platform from side to side, from ceiling to floor. The sight took my breath away.

With the curtain's parting, a rich, deep voice began to tell the story of the crucifixion of Christ, the Lord. My son knew the story, but as it was revealed to him once more, his face glistened with tears in the semidarkness. He took my hand and held it tight, without saying a word. After the story had been told, the curtains were drawn together, then reopened, revealing a large painting depicting Christ's resurrection. After the curtains had closed for the last time, the theater remained darkened for several moments. It was during those heartbeats of time that my son turned to me.

"Why did they kill Him, Mother?" he asked. "I think if He was here now, He would help me. I am good, Mother, I love people. Why don't they love me?" His voice was plaintive with longing.

"They do, dear, they do." I tried to assure him, but the words stuck in my throat, strangling me.

Then he turned to me again. "When I die, do you think They will take *me* in Heaven?" he asked.

"Of course, son, of course." I could hardly get the words out.

As we were leaving the building, Billy turned to me a third and final time and whispered softly, "Then I guess I can wait to be happy."

I was struck to my very soul, and had to struggle to maintain my emotional equilibrium. This very personal, private revelation of my child's agony shook the foundation of my world. I did not share it with anyone; it was too horrifying—that an innocent child should have to look to death as his chance for happiness! *Oh, my son— and oh, my God! Help him.*

I was relieved to get out into the open air. I left with a heavy heart, knowing the depth of my son's pain. The moment of truth had passed.

We thought our next stop should be a complete change of pace from Forrest Lawn, so we went to Disneyland, a treat of pure joy. All during the trip we tried to avoid certain pitfalls. We were discriminating in our choices of entertainment, and avoided loud noisy places. After our troubles at "It's a Small World" at the New York World's Fair we sidestepped The Tiki Room at Disneyland, but saw everything else. We had dealt with a schizophrenic child long enough to know— sometimes—which exposures were safe, and which ones were to be avoided.

Disneyland was a delight to Billy, and so was our trip to San Francisco. We drove along the coastal highway, with its spectacular scenery, up to the Big Sur country. The road hugs the side of the mountains, twisting and turning, with the Pacific Ocean several hundred feet below. We had to drive very carefully as there was nothing between us and the water below—no guard-rails, nothing. A few times, as I drove, I thought my husband was going to jump out of his skin, the road was so hazardous. We rolled along, mile after crooked mile, becoming more and more enthralled with the blue sky and water below. Sometimes we felt we were flying.

Billy loved every mile, as he had always loved the sea, and we couldn't have asked for a better traveling companion. The day was almost gone when we left this highway and arrived in San Francisco by way of monstrous freeways. They provided a harrowing experience—especially since we were not accustomed to the traffic. We had a couple of close calls, and I, for one, was glad when we reached our destination.

We explored the city by cable cars, spending days going up and down hills, until I was becoming sick from the ups and downs. It didn't bother anyone else at all. Billy thought the place was fascinating, especially the boat ride around the bay, under the Golden Gate Bridge, and circling Alcatraz Island Prison. The prison was no longer in use, but Billy insisted on knowing all about it.

"I'm sorry, Billy," I had to confess, "you'll have to ask someone else. I've never been in prison and I don't know anything about it."

So far we had had relatively little trouble with Billy. He had been cooperative and interested in everything. But on our return trip from San Francisco to Los Angeles, he gave us a bad time. We stopped to see San Simeon, the Hearst estate. To get there we had to take a bus up a winding road to the top of a small mountain. On the way up the hill, someone in the bus coughed. From that moment the trip became a nightmare. Billy refused to go with the group. We had to coax him every step of the way. We practically had to carry him. He whined, fussed, hollered, and embarrassed us until I was ready to start screaming myself. The guide talked on and on. We were caught; there was no way back; we had to follow the tour. When it was over, and we returned to our car, my husband and I were exhausted from trying to deal with Billy. Then he started to complain about time. He kept saying *he* couldn't understand the time, and we couldn't understand *him*. He said he was tired, tired, tired. He asked us where we were, though he knew already. He kept this up for a long while, even after we had returned home.

Before we departed, my mother had a farewell dinner for us. One of her guests kept watching Billy pace around before we sat down to eat. Even though he was rather quiet, she asked me what was wrong with him. I told her merely that he was an emotionally disturbed child and did not go into detail. With that she looked at me and said, "Oh! Mother must have been very stern with him when he was a baby."

Her attitude infuriated me, but I should have been used to it by now. People were always drawing the same conclusion without knowing the stupidity it revealed. I didn't enlighten the woman, but charged it up to ignorance. The next day we left.

At the airport, Billy was quiet until we were about to board the plane. He began to pace back and forth, hollering at the top of his voice that he was not going to get on another airplane. We thought he had forgotten his threat. His father finally cornered him and told him *we* were flying home. If he didn't get on the plane he could stay in California without us. We walked away from him. We were both tired of coaxing him.

Billy stopped making a racket and followed us, strapping himself into the seat, but he was not happy about it. As we started to taxi onto the runway he began his loud protesting all over again. I put my arms around him and practically squashed him to keep him in his seat and quiet while we took off.

It was pouring rain when we finally reached Newark

Airport. We had to circle for a long time. Billy was impossible. He kept yelling, "Help! Help! We'll all be killed!" over and over again. I was glad the engine noise was so loud that nobody paid any attention to him. When we touched down on the runway at last, I was a wreck. Before we had taxied to the exit ramp my husband said something to me about what a terrible landing the pilot had made. I hadn't even noticed.

"Never mind about that, Bill," I sighed. "I'm just glad to be back and safe."

We left the plane by the front hatch, and Billy went over to the pilot who was standing near the doorway. "That was a pretty awful landing you made, sir," he said.

"Tell me, son, who told you that?" The pilot looked curiously at him.

"My father," Billy answered. "He used to fly airplanes too."

The man burst out laughing. "Tell your father he was absolutely correct. That was a miserable landing all right."

With that we left the plane. Walking to the main building, I told my husband, "No more long trips with him. I don't think I could take the strain again." I'm sure he felt the same way.

Snug in our home once more, we prepared Billy for the opening of school. I began to see new signs in him that worried me. He grew listless, and at the same time, I sensed his internal tension coming to a full boil. He had had this quality most of his life, but now it was worse than ever. He asked me the same question every day.

"Will *that boy* be in my class again, Mother?" A few days before school opened, he was overwhelmed with anxiety and fear. We tried to assure him things would be different this year, but we just couldn't penetrate the gathering darkness into which he was slipping in his disturbed state of mind.

He had resumed his visits to the psychiatrist upon our return. The psychiatrist did his best to prepare Billy for a better school year, but the child was unmoved by hopes, promises, or any word of encouragement. Because of his attitude, I took him to school the first day and talked to his teacher. Although she was pleasant and interested, I had the feeling that Billy was going to be too rough a customer for her to handle. I spoke to my husband about my feelings, but he said we should give it a chance. The chance was a risky one.

9

We All Died a Little

The sigh of relief I breathed the first day I took Billy to his new class should have stuck in my throat. Because his adversary was not present, I had some hope that things would go better for him. Oh, how wrong I was!

In September his behavior improved somewhat. He was working again, taking some interest in trying to get back into a regular class. He deeply resented us for allowing him to become involved in this special program. I couldn't blame him for his attitude, considering the past year. He wished with all his heart to be with "the regular kids," as he called them. What he failed to realize was that he was not like the regular kids in many ways, but we kept boosting him nevertheless.

"You're doing nicely, dear. Just keep up the good work, and you'll be back in a regular class before you know it. The responsibility rests with you. Daddy and I will do everything we can to help, but you have to do the rest for yourself. We can't go to school for you, Billy." I watched to see how he would take it.

"I know, I know," he sighed. It was an old story to him by now.

I began to see some hopeful signs in Billy. Maybe we *were* on the right track. After all these years of disturbance, there was a momentary lull. Then the inevitable happened. Because there were more pupils, the classes had to be rearranged. And Billy's tormentor was placed in his class.

We were not aware of this transfer right away, but I could see Billy's conduct deteriorating. I was used to this, for it had happened spasmodically as he attended school over the years, but he usually recuperated. This time, the change in him was so radical, it startled me. He came home upset every day, and his limited ability to concentrate diminished to complete inability. He demeaned himself constantly.

"I'm no good. I'm evil, Mother, and I need to be punished," he told me.

"What in heaven's name ever gave you an idea like that?" I asked him. "Stop *saying* such terrible things about yourself! Billy, you're the best and bravest boy I know! Don't say you are evil. You are not!"

"I am, I am, I am!" He screamed and cried, tearing at his hair and pounding his fists against his head as hard as he could. Then he told me the other boy was with him again. My whole being protested against the news.

"You promised me! You promised me he wouldn't be there! You're a liar. I hate you!" Was there no justice for Billy—or for me?

If I tried to explain that the matter was out of our hands, he would be even more furious. So I waited. When he calmed down, and I tried to reason with him, he just looked at me bewildered and confused. He did not understand that his father and I were unable to do anything to help the situation.

Billy's enemy had picked up right where he had left off the year before. Knowing Billy's weaknesses, he took delight in making my son wild. The punching, pinching, spitting, and name calling became a daily routine again. I pitied Billy with all my soul.

"Listen, Billy, you let this boy get away with annoying you to death last year. He's going to keep it up forever—unless you fight back." I knew Billy *couldn't* retaliate but I had to suggest it once more.

He gritted his teeth and hissed through them, "I told you I won't! If I hit him, I'll kill him!" History was repeating itself, and we could see what was coming next. I could not understand why the tormenting was allowed to go *on and on and on.* I could not see what good it did the other child either. He was in that class because he had problems too. I tried to explain this to our son, but I hit a brick wall.

"If he has problems, why does he take them out on me? I wouldn't do that to him."

"Billy, *please, please,* hit him as hard as you can, right in the face." My words sounded ugly. They matched the frustration I felt. "I know we always tell you *not* to do things like that, but you must! You must!" My words were met by torrents of tears, and little else.

After a couple of weeks of this treatment, Billy's suffering was so acute that he began to tear his clothes to shreds in a frenzied effort to escape. Five torn shirts and several overcoat pockets later, we felt we had put up with enough. My husband took the torn shirts to the Assistant Superintendent of Schools. He threw the shirts angrily on the man's desk, demanding to know why a child was permitted to be harassed to the point where he would destroy his clothes.

"Will you please tell me why *nothing* is done to stop the chaotic conduct permitted to go on in that classroom?" Bill demanded. "We were told, when we got involved in this mess, that these classes were set up to help rehabilitate emotionally sick children! If *this* is helping them—" Bill was nearly speechless with mounting fury.

"Mr. Foy, we have other students, and we cannot tailormake a class of one to suit the disabilities of *your* child." The man's apparent calmness was infuriating. "I'm sorry, but that's how it is." He flung out his hands in a gesture of finality.

"In other words, there is nothing you *can* or *will* do about it!" Bill accused him.

"I'm afraid that is the way it is," the man went on. "You know we didn't want to place *your* son in this program to begin with, because of his age." Now they seemed to be blaming us for enrolling him to start with!

My husband came home fed up, and boiling mad.

"All right, Bill, calm down." How ridiculous for me to try to soothe him when I needed soothing myself. "They *haven't* thrown him out yet. But I tell you, if another week goes on like the last one, I am taking him out of school, whether you like it or not. I can teach him myself, and he won't have to go through hell on earth."

"You can't do that, Jessie! It's no good! If he thinks he can escape every time something unpleasant comes along now, he'll do it all his life! He can't spend the rest of his time running away!" It was hard to tell whether Bill was more angry at the school, at Billy, at me, or at his own frustration.

"I know that, but what else can we do?" I begged futilely. "The school certainly isn't going to change the class for us! I just don't know where to turn next," I confessed. "It's driving me mad, watching him suffer."

When my husband, Billy, and I reached the point of no return, I called Billy's psychiatrist and told him I was withdrawing our son from school. I would teach him at home as best I could. Billy could not stand any more punishment.

"Mrs. Foy, don't you realize this is Billy's way of persistently trying to escape from reality, rather than to do anything to cope with it? If you let him establish a pattern, he'll get worse. Keeping him home is no solution either. He'll regress!" The doctor's words were not at all persuasive to me. I had seen too much of Billy's agony.

"Look, doctor, I am aware of all you say, but *we have to live with our son.* The school situation is outrageous! I don't see how *anything* could be *worse* than it is at this moment!"

"Why don't you keep him at home for a while, and then return him? Perhaps a temporary withdrawal would be better than total escape." He was trying to find a satisfactory compromise now. But I was so fed up with the whole mess, I couldn't see any merit in his idea. After fifteen minutes of conversation, he reluctantly agreed to let me withdraw Billy. I was suspicious—I saw residential school looming on the horizon.

When we first noticed the extreme change in our son's conduct and found out about the transfer of his adversary into his class, I called to offer my services as a teacher's helper. I had a college degree, though not in education, and years of practical experience in handling a schizophrenic child. I did not wish to work in my son's class, but in the other group, if they could get someone else to help Billy's teacher maintain order. My idea was ridiculed, and my offer rejected. I was really chagrined when they hired teachers' helpers for this very purpose, *after* we had been forced to withdraw our son from school. For Billy it was *always* too little, too late. I was told a year later that the redheaded menace started to pester another boy after Billy left. This child hit his aggressor so hard in the mouth that he had to go to the hospital for stitches in his cut lip.

Billy's experiences in these two classes set him back years and left deep emotional scars. The tactics used by the school seemed ridiculous to us, and destructive rather than helpful. We were called pests because we wished to protect our child. My husband told me that if he went to the assistant superintendent's office once more, the man would probably throw him out. And so we were on our own.

"Well, Billy, it won't be the first time we've struggled alone," I reminded him. "And something tells me it won't be the last either."

When we withdrew Billy from school, we had asked for a tutor at our home, but the school authorities refused to provide one, although such was the common practice when children were unable to attend regular classes because of some physical disability. They must have felt we were asking for too much, since the class *was* functioning. What they didn't seem to consider was that our son was *not*. At least, that is the impression we got. The Assistant Superintendent of Schools told us a tutor was provided only as a last resort. What did he think our case was?

I began teaching Billy at home for three hours every morning. In the beginning, he was eager to work and did his best for me. Some days he learned quickly; others, I could not penetrate his world. Each day I watched him sink deeper into a state of depression. Shadows' child was consumed with hopelessness. I had to absolutely demand his attention sometimes, by whatever means I could devise. Sometimes he sat crying, telling me he was no good. Then he begged me to help him.

"Help me, Mother, help me!" He screamed until it was all I could do to maintain my self-control. I was

torn asunder, rocked by his fluctuating emotional turmoil and his express desire to learn. Time slipped away,
and he became less communicative. There were still
outbursts of agitation and excitability, when he cursed
his father and me for what we had done to him. He
changed from a rather arrogant adolescent, to a fearful
quaking child, to a screaming infant with a temper tantrum in a short period of time. His fury with us for placing him in those terrible classes was endless. He
couldn't forgive. No amount of explanation would convince him that we had not willed his suffering. His attitude made me think of the unmailed cards he had
written to us when he was away at camp.

As we worked and talked, Billy had a fit if I used certain words he did not like, or that threatened him in
some strange way. Then he would say, "I think I'm
going crazy—out of my mind!"

His thought processes, though never clear and logi-
cal, were becoming so disorganized I had trouble trying
to figure out what he meant by some things he said. As I
had done years before, I pieced his conversations together like puzzles. Besides all this, he adamantly refused to go any place with me during school hours. He
feared people would wonder why he was not in school
himself. Trying to cope with him was shredding our
nerves. Life in our household was intolerable for everyone. Prayer was all that sustained me—almost against
logic I held on to the faith that someday, somehow,
there would be a way. God would have to lead us to it.
On our own, we were lost.

The one thing Billy did not refuse to do was to go to
see his psychiatrist once a week. He told the psychiatrist
all about what was going on at home. He also complained to him of feeling great fatigue. He would lie
down on the couch to rest when they talked. I was

worried that he might be getting diabetes, but he had no other symptoms. The psychiatrist felt his tiredness was due to his pressing emotional problems.

Our visits to the psychiatrist had an established routine. Billy's father would take him to the doctor's office in the morning, and I would pick him up an hour later. One morning I overslept and got downtown late. Billy was nowhere in sight when I arrived, so I ran to the psychiatrist's office to see if he was waiting for me. He wasn't. I returned home by the route I generally took. No Billy. By now I was in a panic. I could not rely on him to remain calm and think straight if I did not show up. My imagination ran wild, thinking of terrible things which might have happened to him. In desperation, I called the police. I asked them to see if they could find him, but warned them not to try to get him into their car. If they saw him, they should call me and tell me where he was. Half an hour later the phone rang. Somehow I had missed him, and he was walking home by our regular route. The officers had asked him his name to make sure they had the right boy. Home at last, he came in from his long walk, cool as a cucumber, but very angry with me.

"Why did you send the police after me?" he demanded.

"I didn't, Billy," I lied. "They probably were wondering why you weren't in school, and stopped to see if they could help you."

I hated to fib, but it saved me hours of accusations and emotional wranglings with him. I was thankful he had found his way home.

One unusual facet of Billy's personality always twisted his father and me into knots. He had an uncanny ability to touch the heart of a problem, even though he was radically disoriented. He knew that something was very wrong with himself.

I remember a perfect example of this. For over a month I had been attending a weekly Bible study course in my church. At the supper table I was discussing an aspect of Christian theology with my husband. The incident had to do with Christ's prayer in the garden of Gethsemane before His betrayal. While He prayed, He asked His Father that "this cup" be passed from Him. If it was not to be passed, He would accept His Father's will. As Christ prayed, his disciples slept. He turned and admonished them for not staying awake. Many Christians believe Christ knew every event in His life beforehand, others do not. The Gethsemane prayer cast some doubt on the validity of the theory that He was all-knowing. My husband and I were discussing our opinions about it. I did not think Billy was listening. He seemed absorbed in thought, and was unusually quiet. Suddenly he turned and looked at his father for a long time, and then at me. Very softly, he said, "Mother, I am like Christ's disciples."

"What do you mean, Billy?" I wanted to know.

"I am failing you, I am failing my father, and I am failing myself! And I don't know why!" His words and expression were full of anguish.

His father turned his face away. I could not look at him either. I was dumbstruck, for with those simple words our son made the saddest confession of human misery and unhappiness I had ever heard! It was so pathetically and clearly said that it tore our hearts out.

"Oh, Billy, dear, you're not failing anyone," his father said lamely.

"Of course not, honey," I chimed in. "We know things haven't been easy for you. But don't worry, it's going to be all right. Have a little faith in yourself and us." How hypocritical I was—talking as if I had any real faith left myself!

When we had assured him as convincingly as we could, I excused myself from the table and went to my room and closed the door. I did not want Billy to hear me crying. I was sick with sorrow for him. How he, a young boy, had borne his own crucifixion all these years was courage itself. How truly brave he was, no one would ever know!

Billy stayed at home with me for the rest of the year. I gave him the best academic instruction I could, working around his emotional problems. They grew worse as he became severely affected by his illness. Things were so bad he was beginning to talk about destroying himself. One night at the supper table, he grabbed a knife and pointed it at his chest, raging at us, "I'll do it! I'll kill myself!"

"Put that knife down at once!" his father yelled back. "Drop it!"

He dropped it, crying, "I can't; I just can't!"

"Of course you can't, and you won't, because we love you, and you love us. You don't want to hurt us, do you!" I wasn't asking a question, I was making an affirmation. But I wasn't sure I was right at all.

When things got beyond Billy's control, he would run into the kitchen, grab a knife from the drawer, and hold it to his chest, hollering that he would "do it." It happened so often, I paid little attention to his threats after a while, except to pray, "God, help him, God, help him," almost automatically. One day, after such a scene, he shot out of the house and wrapped the end of our clothesline around his neck, pulling against one end trying to choke himself. I ran out to remove the line, but his face was almost blue before I could get him untangled. Once, he pulled the same hideous stunt, tottering on stilts. That time, his father rescued him.

The theme of self-destruction permeated the house. I was doing the laundry in the cellar one morning when Billy begged me to help him kill himself. Whenever he talked this way, I tried to dissuade him, to get his mind on something else. This particular day, he was set off by my answer to his question. He grabbed me by the throat with both hands. He was so strong, I had a real struggle extricating myself from his strangling grasp. As I broke free, I slapped him across the mouth as hard as I could.

"Don't you ever do that again!—you hear me? Not ever!" I was shaking with fright and anger. Anger that I could not help him, fright at what we were all becoming!

Billy fell down and started to cry, "I'm sorry! I'm sorry! Please, please, forgive me!" Confession and sorrow poured from him. I reached down and put my arms about him, but I could not speak. This happened early in the day. The very same afternoon he got down on his hands and knees and begged, like a dog, for me to take his life. At that moment, something inside me broke, shattered into a million tiny pieces, and I felt I could not go on another step of life's way. I sent Billy to his room and sat down. My legs were about to collapse under me. I told his father what had happened. We *all* died a little that day.

"Bill, I never thought I'd say this, but I don't think I can go on like this much longer. What are we going to do?" I implored. "I don't want to, but I'm slowly giving up." I didn't acknowledge it aloud; but even my oft-repeated affirmation, "The Lord is my shepherd . . ." had begun to ring hollow in my ears.

"You can't give up—I won't let you!" he shouted. "I know *I* won't, until I close my eyes for good!" Somehow, I felt better, and pulled all my splintered fragments together, determined to work harder than ever to get Billy over his problems. Although I still had deep personal reservations about sending him to residential school, I knew that what we were doing was *not* a solution. The time was approaching for us to consider this final alternative.

His behavior destroyed the last vestiges of outside contact too. Up to this point, he had continued with religious instruction and Y.M.C.A. activities without great difficulty, but now his conduct affected his acceptance in these places too.

One Monday afternoon I drove to pick him up from his religious instruction class, and he did not come out of the building. I waited five minutes before I decided to enter and look for him. I found Billy in the principal's office, crying. The head nun told me he had upset the whole class. As a consequence, the children had ridiculed him, and he had to be removed. She very politely told me she did not think I should bring him back anymore—for *his* sake.

We had a similar experience at the Y.M.C.A. At the end of the season, another boy smacked Billy on his bare bottom with a wet towel in the locker room after swimming. Billy was infuriated by the attack, and became so wild nobody knew what to do with him. The director took Billy in tow and managed to quiet him down, but our son only got into it again in the hallway with the same boy shortly afterward. When Billy's father picked him up that evening, he was politely but firmly told that such outbursts could not be tolerated. The director of young boys' activities implied that he did not wish to see Billy again if he was going to behave in that manner. I never did find out exactly what Billy had done, but it was plainly unacceptable.

Now he was completely alone, with no place to go. He was out of school, out of friends, out of luck. Nobody wanted a problem, large or small. I could not blame them, but it hurt us all the same. The pity was that basically Billy was a very good child, and the loneliness he experienced from constant rejection was pure torture to watch. Granted he wasn't right in mind or spirit, but the loss of human contact, even impersonal contact, overwhelmed him.

If he had not had us at this time, I hate to think of what would have become of him. We loved him so dearly; we always tried to convey to him that he was a fine human being, unique, and he meant the world to each of us. This was not easy, for he resisted any overtures of affection. Everyone had rejected him, and he was not about to trust or have faith in even his parents or close relatives. I longed to get close to him emotionally, to comfort him, but his invisible wall stood between us. He was now truly Shadows' child, not ours, not the world's.

10

Victory Through Surrender

Billy finally had a second neurological examination, including an E.E.G., the first having been done when he was six years old. The second examination revealed a possible brain disfunction syndrome, resulting in so-called hyperkinetic behavior. Billy's hyperactivity had been obvious for some time. The results of the E.E.G. were only midly abnormal, minimal in fact.

"It's not unusual enough to be concerned about," the doctor assured us.

Then why did you mention it at all? I wondered. It was still a worry to me in spite of the doctor's insistence that the child was not brain damaged, as he originally suspected. To us, the possible brain disfunction syndrome was another distressing diagnosis piled up on all the rest.

Complicated as his symptoms became, and hard as he was to manage during this disorganized year, Billy still tried to keep up with some work. After I removed him from class in November, 1965, the months rolled by with no action by the Board of Education on our request for a tutor. We decided that they felt Billy should be in a residential school. It was obvious that they were not going to aid us further until we were forced to the same conclusion.

Billy's father and I talked to his psychiatrist about the whole situation, and he wasn't very encouraging. He felt that Billy had reached the residential school stage. We had tried everything. Nothing worked. We could not fight the whole school system any longer. Maybe we *were* wrong, and they were right. Perhaps a therapeutic environment *would* do the trick. His father felt it might help, but I harbored grave doubts.

Although I hated the whole idea of a residential school for Billy, I had to admit we were in real trouble with him at home. Still, the thought of sending him away made me sick. The fear that arose inside me when I thought of releasing my son to the indifferent care of someone else for an indeterminate period of time gave me the horrors. I felt angry at my own inadequacy to help him. I felt guilty that I could not reach down inside him and tear out the darkness from his soul. Love, our prayers, our deep devotion to him—nothing seemed to be enough, no matter how we tried to help him. But what could strangers do for him that we could not, with good outside help? The psychiatrist explained that Billy would have daily therapy and be with other boys in a good and different atmosphere. I agreed that therapy might help. The different atmosphere might be helpful too. But other boys? No. They hadn't proved helpful to Billy before. Nevertheless, we would try to find a proper residential school. Billy's doctor had warned us, "It's either residential school, or we lose him entirely and forever." My back was against the wall. I succumbed to their judgment and will.

Against my intuitive judgment, which was not infallible, we began to search. We wrote and visited schools from Massachusetts to California and Texas in our efforts to find one appropriate for Billy, and one we could afford. This quest was an education in itself! Several of the schools we visited had physical facilities so depressing they would have made a normal individual ill to reside in them. Many were overcrowded, dirty, and so malodorous I had to go outside to avoid nausea. One place in Connecticut looked like a disordered pigsty, inside and out. There was everything imaginable strewn about. The residents were allowed to smoke and do almost anything else they desired. The ages of the boys there varied, but they all lived together. Billy was twelve and I was afraid he might be influenced to pick up undesirable habits.

The attitude of the instructors and attendants in many places was unconcerned and permissive. Unfeeling and cruel attitudes expressed by the staff in other schools were appalling. We were told in one reputable school that all the children's papers were marked correct, even if everything the child did was wrong. The idea was to build the child's confidence.

"What happens when the patient leaves and continues to do his work wrong in another school situation?" I asked the principal. "Wouldn't it be twice as hard to relearn all the work over again correctly?" I was genuinely concerned. The principal didn't answer my question. He just shrugged his shoulders as if to say, "Who cares?" We were flabbergasted.

The same principal said that when a child became upset in class he was sent about the school to empty wastepaper baskets—the old "chop the wood" routine, to get something out of your system. We had used this same technique on Billy at home.

We continued to write letters to every facility we could consider. The results were discouraging. Most schools had long waiting lists, two years or more minimum. Many urged us to let our local community handle the problem. Apparently they had missed the substance of our letters. All the school brochures looked promising when we read them, and we became hopeful. It was when we dug below the surface that we discovered the real truth. In most instances, all they offered was a change of scene. Some were trying to do a decent job, but their financial resources were limited, restricting their ability to obtain staff with sufficient training.

The fees for the residential placement of an emotionally disturbed child or adult ranged from five thousand dollars to twenty thousand dollars a year, with no guarantees! After months of looking, talking, and writing, we found a school in a neighboring state that seemed well-run and appropriate for our son's needs.

Our initial inquiries began in December, 1966, with the approval of Billy's psychiatrist. He had two other patients, sicker than our son, who had attended this institution. Both of them had made very satisfactory adjustments and were now functioning on their own.

We wrote to the school, giving a general outline of our son's case. We also gave written permission to all Billy's doctors to submit their findings to the school. The more involved I became in all this, the more I hated the whole idea; but I was not in a position to do anything else. I was worried about my husband, and had to regard his feelings too, so my hands continued to be tied. For months, while we were going through all this, he had been literally living on sleeping pills. We had been at each other's throats over our son's welfare. Sometimes it had been so bad, we felt our marriage disintegrating under the tension. Billy's handicap had imposed a discipline upon us that was unbearable at times. It left scars on all of us, but we had a mutual bond: anything, everything, humanly possible, must be done for this child. And the responsibility had to be ours.

The preliminary steps for an application to a residential school of this type take quite a while. In the meantime, the local Board of Education was providing nothing in the way of educational help for Billy. They seemed to be oblivious of their legal obligation to try to educate our child under the Beadleston Act of the State of New Jersey. My husband hammered at their door until, finally, they acted.

We received a letter to the effect that they would not return our son to their special class. What a joke that was! We did not want him returned, especially now that we had decided on residential schooling for Billy. This was in March, 1967. We had originally requested a tutor in November, 1966. In the same letter we were told that a tutor would be provided until Billy was accepted elsewhere. It was a little better than nothing at all.

When the tutor arrived, she quickly found that Billy wasn't easy. If he was responsive, they did well together. If he was not, she left work to be done, and I would see that he did it. I kept hearing the echo, "Leave the teaching to the teachers." We all did the best we could, and lived in the hope that real help would soon be forthcoming. Meanwhile, we continued to negotiate with the local board.

Under the Beadleston Act, if no local facility is available, the Board of Education must look outside its own limits for a proper program to meet a child's needs. In our case, we had done the looking for them, but they were still financially responsible—within limits—for the educational portion of the cost of keeping Billy in a residential school. The school, of course, had to meet their standards for approval. Our application to the school had to be approved at the county level too, for it is the county board that reimburses the local board for their expenditures in the child's behalf. Since the school was going to cost us $15,000.00 a year, we were greatly appreciative of any financial subsidy we could obtain.

Billy needed help right then and there, but it seemed to take forever for all the interviews and paper work. While we waited, we kept Billy going, mentally and physically. If we had not, I am sure we would have lost him forever. Not only was he ill, but he had been bounced from one ghastly situation to another, enough to discourage a perfectly normal child. For the first time, he was giving up trying. He felt completely hopeless, useless. He told me so every day. He said he would be that way until he died. I nearly broke down, listening to him, and so did his father. We kept telling him about the residential school, and he held on by a spider's thread, hoping they could help him. He desperately wanted help, despite the fact that he sometimes denied it.

It was a torturous year for all of us. Billy's dad and I were running out of hope, but we never let him know it. We were so sick ourselves, that we quarreled over him constantly, usually late at night, after he had fallen asleep. We had no rest, no peace, no harmony, each of us suffering his own personal defeats, and simultaneously working to prevent our only child from becoming an emotional basket case. Sometimes I wished, with all my soul, to run away, to die—anything to escape. His father felt the same way, but we could not desert our son. Escape was only wishful thinking. We were going around in circles worrying already, and then I began to worry for an added reason.

Billy had started to eat constantly. He was using food as a substitute for companionship. He was getting heavy —not fat, but above his normal weight—and I could not stop him. I was tempted to put a lock on the refrigerator door, as every time I turned my back, he was swinging it open. His eating did not give him satisfaction in the true sense of the word; rather, it was a compulsive act he could not control. As I watched him go from one odd thing to another, I kept praying we would hear from the school soon!

One day we were invited to visit one of their units. While there, we were encouraged to ask questions and we did.

"I am very much interested in finding out what type of emotional help you give these boys," I said. "It is our understanding that what you do is on a daily basis." I wanted to make sure my understanding was correct this time.

"That is not quite correct, Mrs. Foy," our interviewer explained. "Therapy is given on a priority basis; that is, the most troubled patients see the psychiatrist three times a week, the less complicated twice a week, and some of the children receive no therapy at all." His answer was disappointing to me, but at least it sounded honest.

"This was not what we were led to believe," my husband objected. "But I guess three times a week is better than what we are doing now." At that moment neither of us knew anything else to do for Billy. We'd have to accept what they offered and make the best of it.

In April, 1967, all the necessary reports had been filed with the residential school. Our local Child Study Team had visited the school and put their stamp of approval on Billy's application so that we would receive financial help. The last thing to be done was to furnish them with the complete, comprehensive report of Billy's psychiatrist. When that had been done, we were all asked to appear for a final two-day evaluation. The first steps were no guarantee that our son would be accepted. The fee for the two-day interview was $75.00. This was a standard practice at most facilities, and the fee was not refunded even if the child was not accepted for enrollment. One could easily spend a small fortune having applications refused! Our interviews were to take place in their main offices, and we would have to stay overnight.

While we were waiting to learn the date of our appointment, we spent our time preparing Billy for a long separation from us in the event he was accepted. The day, April 24, came at last. We had been asked to bring a supply of clothes along for Billy. Just before we left home, Billy's psychiatrist assured us our son would be one of their better patients. He had no conception of the calamity awaiting us.

Something kept buzzing around in my head on the long drive out of our state. I kept remembering two visitors I had recently had in my home, and what they had said to me. One of the visitors was Billy's priest. The other was my minister.

For the last few months Billy had *not* been going to Sunday school, but he *did* believe in God, and he wanted to be confirmed. The priest felt he could help him, but he did not want Billy to believe that confirmation would solve all his problems. He had the feeling, from talking to Billy, that he was counting on God's grace to fulfill his longing to be well—and that he expected his confirmation to be the time when God would immediately restore him to perfect health. The priest did not have that kind of faith. He felt it would be tragic for Billy to be confirmed and, necessarily, disappointed. After that visit, the priest never came back to see our son.

My own minister told me the same thing. He came to the house one dismal, gray day. I didn't know him well, for I had only recently transferred my membership to his church. I explained to him about Billy as well as I could. It was not easy. When I had finished, he said,

"Jessie, you and your husband have done everything humanly possible for your child. God does not ask any more. If this new school you have told me about cannot help, then you must accept His Will in peace."

"But that's the whole point, Reverend!" I told him. "I cannot accept the fact that there is nothing more we can do. I don't believe it is ever God's will for one of His little ones to suffer. *He* wants Billy well, *more* than I do. I do feel helpless sometimes, but I can't stop hanging on to the thought that there may be something we've overlooked."

He nodded, apparently content to leave it that way, and shook my hand. "So be it then, and if I can help you, please call on me." With that he had left. We were to talk again, many times. He was always consoling, always encouraging, always helpful.

When we reached our destination, I stopped my thinking about my conversations with Bill's priest and my minister. We were taken into an office, where we waited until one of the foundation's social workers was free to talk to us.

Billy was his usual nervous self, but he calmed down slightly when the woman entered the room. During the course of the interview, Billy's father and I were talking. At one point his dad said something Billy did not like. Billy lunged at him, grabbing his shirt. "Are you making fun of me?" he demanded.

Alarm registered on the woman's face. I watched her mouth drop. "Oh, my goodness! He isn't violent, is he?" she asked. She seemed horrified.

"Oh, no, heavens no." I tried to make light of the incident. "He's just on edge—and nervous," I told her, feeling more than a little nervous myself. She cast a strange glance my way. I didn't intend to tell her about the time Billy nearly strangled me. Still, it was obvious she didn't believe my protestation. Then she proceeded to make some comment about the way he walked. "Oh, I *like* that gait! I just *love* the way you walk!" she gushed at Billy. "Oh, *isn't that cute!*" She was almost clapping her hands. I could have thrown up! But I said nothing. Next, Billy was taken to see one of their psychologists, while Bill and I were left with the social worker to discuss Billy's future.

My husband began the conversation. "We have brought our son to you in the hope that you will be able to help him where we have failed," he admitted. "It is our sincere wish that we will not have to take him home again. We have tried everything we know to help him. There are only three things left that could be wrong— his environment, a genetic defect, or some chemical disorder we are unaware of." He paused for a moment.

"What you have mentioned is only a small portion of the whole picture," our interviewer replied.

In other words, us, I thought. I had been conditioned to stay on the defensive.

"If a proper environment and school *don't* help," Bill broke in, "there is only one thing left as far as I can see —and that's a hospital." I always cringed at that eventuality.

"What makes you think this is not the case already?" the caseworker asked, adding to my fears. Her presumptuousness made my skin crawl. She continued to ask us questions, frequently repeating the one about whether or not Billy was violent. She must have suspected that I was not telling the whole truth. Soon she launched her attack on me, watching intently for any over-reaction to her probing questions.

"Mrs. Foy, is it true that you were the one who insisted that Billy have orthodontic work done?"

"Yes, I was," I answered proudly.

"May I ask if you were aware that any work involving body openings could have deep emotional complications for a child?" *Was she accusing me of something?*

"I don't know about complications," I said, without hesitation, "but I do know that having Billy's teeth straightened was less trouble to all of us than almost anything else we went through with him. He was absolutely wonderful about it, and wanted it done himself," I answered, justifying my action still further. By that time I was becoming quite angry.

Continuing on her unalterable course, the social worker said she had read all the reports sent to the school concerning our son's past.

"I'm considered quite good at reading between the lines." She raised her eyebrows significantly at me, "Especially between the lines of school psychologists' reports." According to her, the psychologist's report on Billy implied that we were blaming all our problems on Billy's teachers. I felt that was simply ridiculous! She ended her interview with a final word about our son's behavior: "Very bizarre, you know!"

My head was about to burst with aching, and I kept thinking to myself, *Are these people real? Are we making application to join a country club? Can they be genuinely interested in trying to help sick children?*

Billy had been returned to us after a twenty minute interview with one of their psychologists. I thought twenty minutes was too short a time for a thorough examination. We were told to bring Billy back the next day, not to those offices, but to one of their units in the country, for their final decision. We returned to our motel and didn't say much to each other. Each of us was wrapped up in private thoughts. When Billy was asleep, my husband said to me, "They're not going to take him." Inwardly I agreed, but did not say so out loud. I thought I'd reserve judgment till the final hour. It would soon be upon us.

The next morning we drove for miles into the country. The unit there was beautiful, built in a modern style, clean, and pleasing to the eyes. Billy went for an educational evaluation, and the attending psychiatrist observed him part of the time. Bill and I waited in the reception room. Forty-five minutes later the social worker appeared and invited us into the psychiatrist's office.

The psychiatrist stood up and began to pace around as he told us that they had many children sicker than our son in residence. "The ways in which these other children handle their problems, however," he stopped to clear his throat, "make it far easier to treat them than it would be to treat Billy." He explained to us that theirs was not a closed system. "There are no locks, gates, or guards to keep the children in." Here he paused significantly.

I looked at my husband just then and watched his ordinarily ruddy complexion turn the color of death. I could imagine what he was thinking.

Proceeding again, the psychiatrist said he felt our son needed "constant supervision in a hospital." Then he added, "Perhaps someday, someone can get at the roots of Billy's deep emotional problems." I tried to swallow. He made "someday" sound like "never."

He was alarmed, he said, at the child's apparent deterioration, considering the original information he had received on all of Billy's reports. Listening to him, I thought, *He's talking about a thirteen-year-old boy! My God! Who is he to judge so quickly?* I thought too, that I would faint from the surge of weakness that flooded me. Glancing at my husband, I saw that he was having a similar reaction to the man's words.

Then the social worker entered the conversation

again. She told us she was an "expert at opening hospital doors—preferably a state hospital in Billy's case." She told us there was no longer any stigma attached to hospital treatment for emotional illness. She further related that she had known families who had spent all their financial resources in private institutions, without results. She sounded falsely sympathetic as she concluded condescendingly, "Perhaps your psychiatrist has put you through all these preliminary steps looking for a residential school, to prepare you for something else."

I finished that sentence in my own mind—*hospital confinement.* And my blood boiled. This was my own flesh she was so easily talking about, not some inanimate object! I was so furious, I didn't know which way to look. There was so much I wanted to say, but for once, I was speechless.

Billy's father picked up the conversation. He told them politely that we had not come for a psychological education regarding our son's condition; we had come for help for him, and we were willing to pay for it. He told them the picture they were painting did not correspond with the opinion of Billy's pscychiatrist, who had known Billy since he was five years old. Bill explained how he had questioned our doctor many times about the advisability of hospital treatment for Billy. The psychiatrist had always told us he would inform us immediately if he felt it necessary to put Billy in a hospital.

Mercifully, our son was not present when all this was going on, and before we were dismissed, I exploded. In shocked anger I stood up and shouted at both of them: *"GO TO HELL!"* It wasn't very ladylike, but I *had* to get it out of my system. I had heard enough! No child of *ours* was going to rot his life away in some hospital until *someone, someday,* got around to finding out what was causing his problems—not as long as we had life in our bodies!

When we picked Billy up on our way out of the building, he asked us several times if he was going to stay there. I couldn't answer him. I just drew him close as we walked to the car. The long ride home was pure torture. I couldn't look at my husband, and he didn't say much except to answer Billy's questions. The look of disappointment on the child's face was eloquent. He, too, realized this was his last chance, and he asked me repeatedly, "Why don't they want me there, either, Mother?"

It was too pitiful to bear. When I was able to speak I answered, "I'm sorry, Billy, but they had so many others that there is no room right now. They have to take the others first." He accepted my answer, but I could see he was terribly hurt.

When we pulled into the driveway of our home, my husband got out of the car and went into the house. He entered the bedroom and locked the door behind him without a word. I could hear him sobbing and left him alone. In all the years we had been married, I had never heard him cry, nor had I seen him falter, even under killing strain. I felt a compassion for him I had never known before. He had reached *his* breaking point. I knew he would recover, but right now his pain was mine. I gave him the solitude he needed.

I took Billy outside to help me unload the car, keeping his mind and hands busy. I did not want him to hear his father. When he asked me where his dad was, I said, "Look, honey, it was a very long ride home, and I think Daddy went to take a nap. He was tired!" After that, I don't know how I managed, but we did get through the rest of the day.

When Billy was out of earshot, I called his psychiatrist and told him what had happened. He was aghast. He asked me why they did not call him if they had any questions after observing our son. I couldn't answer, except to say that they had already made up their minds not to take him. A call would have done no good.

Bill finally came out of the bedroom, and we ate supper in inarticulate sorrow! When I saw the aching despair in his eyes, I felt shaken to my soul. He had always been my rock in time of deep trouble. Now we were both sick in body and spirit.

As all things do, the day finally ended, and we went to bed—Bill with his sleeping pills, I to toss and think and worry. I could not take a sleeping pill—they always made me sick, and I felt terrible enough already.

Lying there, I realized how we had been torn asunder by the day's revelations! All hope of saving our child's life was washed away in a monstrous tide of "the considered opinions of others." We were dashed cruelly against the jagged rocks of complete helplessness, shattered and bleeding, without hope, without a prayer. Every door was closed, every hope of escape destroyed, each flickering light extinguished with words of discouragement.

Why? I asked myself. *What has our poor, sad, Shadows' child done to deserve this tragedy? What will happen to him after we are gone? Who is there to care?* I questioned myself relentlessly. Billy had courageously fought this Devil's plague against unbelievable odds; but he was on the verge of losing the battle, and so were we.

I must have been awake for hours, thinking, searching, when I felt something—an unseen force—drawing me. I had been tossing over and over on my bed like a roast cooking on a spit, for what seemed like forever. Suddenly I stopped and listened to the rhythmic breathing of the others in the house. Slipping quietly from my bed, I put on my robe and walked from the silent house into our yard. I sensed an inner Presence and fell to my knees on the cold ground, praying to God for my son's salvation.

Bereft of human comfort there in the still darkness, I turned to the last refuge of hope—my Lord, Jesus—

Consumed in a loneliness only the broken-hearted know, I asked Him for help. Remembering my minister's words, I promised to try to accept His Will. I do not know how long I remained under the canopy of brilliant stars, but I cried until there were no tears left. I was exhausted! The anguish of my being was crushing me, but somehow, as I prayed, I could not let go or allow myself to give in to self-pity and failure. I knew that nothing but death itself would turn us from our goal to have our child complete and well. For surely his wholeness *was* God's will too!

Eventually I rose, grateful for the shielding privacy the night had offered, and returned to my bed, conscious of possessing internal peace. I slept undisturbed for the first time in years. I had hope, though I knew there really was none, and I knew I would always feel this way. I had found the peace that passes understanding, His peace.

Today, when I think of that night and hear others belittle the power of prayer, I remember my blessed gift. It was as if I myself had been resurrected by my loving Father. And I thanked my God.

"I sought the Lord, and he heard me and delivered me from all my fears." (Psalm 34:4)

11

A Ray of Hope

The day after our return from disaster, my husband went to inform the Assistant Superintendent of Schools that Billy's application had been rejected. As crushed as we then felt about the whole affair, we were soon to be grateful for their refusal to take him. Anyhow, Bill admitted to the man that we were defeated for the moment, but that we would not stay that way. At the time I could not see how we were going to recover, but I did know that all things change. I was counting on that. The Assistant Superintendent said that the Child Study Team would continue to seek another possible placement for our son. In the interim, they would send the tutor to finish the 1967 school year.

For days I walked around in a state of emotional emptiness, worrying about Billy. How we managed to function, I don't remember. Inwardly, I knew that whatever our burden, God would give us the strength to bear it, but I still had seizures of great doubting. When my family tried to console me, it only made matters worse. I could not listen to them. Billy's father and I just stopped talking about things for a little while. Silence seemed the best solution, at least temporarily, but one persistent and agonizing question remained: "Where and why had we failed him?"

One evening I went to visit a friend, just to get out of the house. I wasn't in a socializing mood, but I needed fresh air and a change for a few hours. I had not seen my friend for a while, and she asked me how we had fared at the school. I told her what they had said about our son. Then I broke down and cried, something I loathe to do in front of anyone. I did not realize it at the time, but in the next few minutes my prayers were answered. God was indeed working in mysterious ways.

My friend began to tell me about a television program she had watched, and although she did not know the exact nature of Billy's illness, she said that what was discussed was very interesting and might be helpful to Billy.

"Jessie, it was the Allen Burke Show—you know the one I mean—I'm sure you've watched it sometime yourself," she said. I acknowledged that I had.

"Tell me about it," I told her, and then asked, "What makes you think it would help Billy?"

"Well, a Dr. Hoffer was on the show, discussing a new and effective treatment for schizophrenics. It had something to do with giving these people massive doses of vitamins."

"Vitamins?" I wasn't sure I had heard correctly. "What kind of vitamins?"

"It's called the megavitamin treatment," she said, "and it's based on B-3 and C, niacin and ascorbic acid. If I understood the man, schizophrenics are lacking an enzyme, and these vitamins combine in the system to help form the missing substance—something like the way you diabetics take insulin to make up for the lack of it. He says the patients' adrenal glands don't function properly, and that so far, this is the most effective treatment they have found. Why don't you look into it? Maybe it will help."

I couldn't be hopeful just then, but let her talk on.

"They also told about how this Dr. Hoffer and a Dr. Humphrey Osmond had written a book called *How to Live with Schizophrenia.*" I must not have been reacting at all, just nodding dully at her. She seemed a little bit impatient with me.

"For goodness' sakes, Jessie! Why don't you at least get the book and read it? What have you got to lose?" She had me there, I had to admit. It couldn't be *too* much trouble. But really she was still not getting through to me completely.

"Why don't we talk about something else?" I pleaded. "Let's drop the subject. I came over to get away from it. Just leave me alone with my misery. After all these years, I am afraid to do any more wishing." How quickly I had given up the perfect peace He had given me!

But my friend did not give up easily, bless her; and as she kept on chatting, I felt a stirring in my memory. A lost thought came forth and rang a bell; then the bell tolled. Of course! I had heard about this same treatment through a radio broadcast, about a year before. How could I have forgotten? I had even asked Billy's psychiatrist to look into it for me. He had reported that there wasn't much to it, so I had dismissed it from my mind. I was feeling so low this evening that I totally rejected the idea of vitamin therapy for what was supposed to be a mental illness allegedly caused by us. Hadn't we been informed by all the experts that it had been caused by us? What else were we to believe? And how could vitamins help? No, it was too farfetched.

I went home and to bed, but my friend's words played on my mind like a phonograph, over and over, as I attempted to sleep. I began to wonder. *Is there a chance? Are there possibilities despite what Billy's psy-*

chiatrist said a year ago? Maybe? Perhaps? Suppose it really would work! All at once I was desperate. I had to *know!*

The next morning I got busy. First I called the television station that had presented the program. They gave me the name of Dr. Hoffer's and Dr. Osmond's publisher and I called them, after first ordering their book. The publisher suggested I call the Princeton Neuropsychiatric Institute in New Jersey where Dr. Osmond was director. Dr. Osmond's personal secretary was most helpful. I asked her if the megavitamin treatment had merit, for I was not about to start working my way up another blind alley. She said it *did* work but warned me that it takes time, in some cases a very long time. *What was time to me?* I thought. Time was about all I had left. She gave me the names of two psychiatrists who used this treatment. One was in Trenton, the other in New York City. We lived closer to New York, and I decided to call this man for an appointment. It could do no harm. It might even help where nothing else had.

Since our return from our two-day interview in April, Billy had begun to balk at seeing his local psychiatrist. I think he knew he was nearing the end of the line. He had given up trusting or trying. This was the worst of it; because previously, no matter how black events had been, he had kept on wishing to be better. Now he said nothing about being better—ever.

When I made my decision to experiment with vitamin therapy, I called Billy's psychiatrist and told him what I planned to do. He said little, but wished me good luck and added that he would be interested in Billy's progress. As soon as I finished talking to him, I reached the other psychiatrist in New York. I explained a little of our son's background to him, and he agreed to see the child the latter part of May, 1967. I suppose it might have been more sensible to read the book first. Maybe I was putting the cart before the horse, but by now I was determined to keep my son out of a hospital by any means I could find. We had reached the court of final appeal, and our son's whole life was at stake.

The book arrived, and I brought it home, placing it on a table in the den. It had a black cover with the title word, *Schizophrenia,* written in bold yellow letters. The word was split in half, with a space in the center dividing each letter. Billy came into the room, picked up the book, and stared at the title for a few seconds. He put it down again, turning to me, saying very seriously, "That's what I am, Mother. I am that word, split, going in two different directions at once."

I couldn't believe my ears. I knew he had not heard or seen the written word before. I had just been told that my child was relatively hopeless, and here he demonstrated a perception and a directness that were absolutely remarkable. Besides this insight, he also knew that he could not go on much longer the way he felt and acted. The thoughts of his future frightened him. This was our real sadness. To be ill and unaware is one thing. To be ill without hope—this is tragedy. I could not let it happen—not to Billy.

While I was making arrangements to start his new treatment, I kept my actions a secret from my husband until everything was set. It wasn't that I was afraid to try it, but I knew he had almost given up. He came in from work a few days later, and I related to him all the steps I had taken. He nearly hit the ceiling.

"What the hell do you think you're doing? Where do you get off at making a decision like that without telling me first?" He was furious! "The kid is messed up enough, and now you're going to start fouling up his body chemistry. Have you lost your sanity? No, absolutely no! I won't hear of it! Now you call that doctor up and cancel that appointment."

I had purposely postponed telling him, as this was what I expected him to say. He raved on for ages, but I did not listen.

"I tell you, Bill, I will not cancel that appointment, and I don't care what you say—I am going through with it." I had never been more determined—about anything. "What else have we got? I don't care if you hit me, I am not going to do what you say and that's that!" I would not let him outshout me.

"You have made most of the important decisions," I went on, "and I am making this one, like it or lump it. I have listened to your reasoning for years. Now I am going to try something on my own. You don't have to accept the responsibility for anything that happens if it doesn't work. And I'll pay for it myself." I was screaming! "But I'm telling you right now, you are expected to go with me for the first visit!"

That did it. He started hollering at me all over again.

"Go *with* you? Listen, madam-know-it-all, if this treatment is so damn good why haven't we heard about it before? Why aren't the other psychiatrists using this treatment?" Then *I* hit the roof!

"I don't care why other psychiatrists are not using vitamins to treat their patients. Nothing that they *have* used has helped our son, and that's all I am interested in." I was glaring ferociously at him. "I tell you what; *you* don't *have* to come with me. You don't have to do anything but stay out of it entirely. The outcome will be on my head. Now shut up!"

We had a real fight going but I wasn't going to give an inch. I didn't care what he said—or what he did. If the house had fallen in on us, I would not have budged.

Bill condescended to read the book, after our

tempers cooled. He grudgingly admitted the vitamin treatment might have a slight chance, but told me not to count on it. In the end, his analyzing scientific mind took over, and he admitted that the caliber of the men who had written the book was such that he could not discount their opinions without further evidence. We couldn't go down any further; the only way left was up.

Our heated argument took place at the beginning of May, 1967. We had to wait until the 31st for our first appointment. During these days Billy stayed at home with me. His tutor did what work she could with him each school day for one hour. I did what I could with him, too. Once in a while, I told him about this new approach to his illness, but not too often, for I did not want him to be disappointed again.

To fill in the gap of contact with the outside world, for he now refused to go anywhere with me, his father decided to buy a small boat. Even though he would not talk to strangers, we felt he should be out in the air and sunshine where there were others about, or he would lose contact with everything. With the boat, we had someplace to take him on the weekends. It worked very well.

May 31st came, and my husband, unthrilled and still disgruntled, went with us to New York. He was a hard man to convince. While Bill and I gave our son's history to the doctor, Billy interrupted our conversation incessantly, interjecting minutely detailed explanations of everything we talked about. He frequently leaned over the doctor's desk to emphasize a point, then retreated behind our chairs to pace back and forth like a caged animal clawing to escape his prison. He pounded his fists together as he walked. He told the psychiatrist he needed "food, drink, education, and protection," and in the next breath, he threatened to be like Hitler and destroy the world and everything in it if no one helped him.

"Well, Billy, your parents will provide you with food, drink, education, and protection, and we will take care of the rest. That's why they have brought you to me," the psychiatrist explained quietly. But even after that reassurance, Billy raged and had outbursts of yelling. Trying to ignore the commotion he created in the background, Billy's father and I continued asking the doctor questions.

Bill started with, "Will you please tell me why all the other psychiatrists aren't using this megavitamin treatment for schizophrenics if it really works? You see, to me it doesn't make sense that so few can be right and the others all wrong."

The psychiatrist didn't seem at all insulted by his question, but answered it matter-of-factly. "Mr. Foy, at the present time not all psychiatrists are ready to accept the bio-chemical approach to emotional disorders, but it is coming. I think they are waiting to be certain that it works for all, before they use or endorse it. I have had considerable success with the treatment, especially with early diagnosis. The sooner the treatment is started— especially with children—the more effective it can be." He made us no promises and warned that it takes time. Because of the long duration of the illness in our son's case, he felt his chances might be less promising than some. He was honest, and for this, I liked the man instantly.

"Do you think that it is possible for a child to be born with the illness?" I asked. He nodded affirmatively. I felt this was true of Billy, for he had been difficult from the very beginning. I asked the psychiatrist another question: "How will we know if the vitamins are doing Billy any good?"

He smiled, and said, "You'll know"; and then went on, "At the present time we are learning more about the illness, but the tools we have to work with are limited. The vitamins, a few drugs, shock treatments, psychotherapy—that's about it." He prescribed the vitamins for Billy and told us he would like to see him again in a month's time.

Billy started taking the pills on June 8, 1967. Suddenly, he developed an urgent desire to be well. He told us he would do anything and everything to feel better, and he meant it. His attitude helped him take the required large number of pills each day. They went down without a whimper. The strength of the vitamins was far above a normal vitamin dosage, but he had no difficulty or ill effects from them.

When we returned to the doctor a month later, I took Billy alone. The psychiatrist told me to double the vitamin dose. He also added another of the B vitamins, and a drug that was supposed to bring more oxygen to the child's brain. He encouraged me to continue the treatment for a minimum of two years in Billy's case. Since the child had been ill for thirteen years, I felt two years would be a reasonable trial. On my return home, my husband questioned me carefully.

"Are you sure he said *double* the dosage?" he asked, incredulous. "That seems like an awful lot of pills to me. I don't think Billy can handle that many!" Bill shook his head.

I didn't want to discuss it further.

"That's what the man said, and if he wants me to give him that many, I intend to do it." End of conversation!

From the time he started to take the pills until they were doubled, we noticed no difference in Billy at all. He continued to speak poorly, act strangely, and always seemed ready to jump out of his own skin. A short time following the doubling of the dose, we saw a radical switch in Billy's behavior.

He began to speak to us in a completely clear and normal manner, with none of his usual hang-ups, repetitions, silliness, or other oddities present in his speech. The topics of his conversations were intelligent. His hyperactivity stopped. He gave up asking or talking about killing. When he spoke, his thought patterns were uninterrupted; and his attitudes had changed unbelievably—all within two or three days. Mr. Hyde became Dr. Jekyll!

A few days later, in late July, we were spending an evening on our boat. Billy began to complain. "I don't feel well, I'm sick. I want to go home."

"What do you mean, Billy? Do you feel physically sick? Or are you upset about something?" I asked him.

"My stomach hurts. Take me home!" He was becoming boisterous. We had all we could do to keep him quiet. He grumbled at the top of his lungs. Rather than try to treat him there or stifle his outcries, we packed up and headed for home. This was nothing new to us—we had done it many times before. On the way home we had to stop several times. Billy was vomiting, and I thought he might be sick from a virus, but he had no fever.

We got him into bed at home, where he was deathly ill, vomiting continuously all night. My husband started berating me for poisoning the kid with "those damn pills."

"Will you please be quiet while I call the doctor?" I implored. He wasn't quiet. I tried several times to reach the doctor the next morning and for the next three days; but he was on vacation and I could not get him. So, I took it upon myself to stop the medication completely. When I finally did contact the doctor, he agreed with my husband that the pills had undoubtedly poisoned the child. He told me to reintroduce them slowly, working up the the original prescribed dosage.

He recovered from the poisoning, but his improvement slowed down tremendously. It was very subtle, but he was changing.

Because he was generally so much better, my two aunts decided to take Billy and his cousin on a trip to Expo 67 in Canada. The morning they left it was raining heavily, and I tried to persuade them to postpone their trip a day. Driving conditions were very poor, and I wanted to relieve my own anxiety for their safety, but they started out on Thursday morning. After their departure, my husband and I headed for our boat. We needed a few days of rest and relaxation. On Monday we received a call from one of my aunts. I was thinking to myself as I headed for the telephone, *What now? I might have known it would be something!* I picked up the receiver and asked, "What's the matter with Billy?"

"I really don't know," my aunt replied, "but he is miserable. He has been driving us crazy, complaining that he is getting sick. But I can't see anything wrong with him. He says his throat is dry, so we brought him home, I drove all night to get him here." She sounded exhausted.

"We're on our way," I said, and hung up.

We left the shore and headed for my sister's house, where everyone was sleeping, catching up after their midnight ride. We let Billy sleep too, but when he woke up, we discovered that the mucous membranes of his nose, mouth, and throat were indeed dry. No wonder he was suffering and uncomfortable! Too much vitamin C! Now I was beginning to speculate on the wisdom of these massive doses of the substances the doctor recommended. I called him again. We lowered the vitamin C gradually until he had no further ill effects from it and eventually reached a fairly stabilized dose.

Except for these two upsets, Billy continued to improve—but at a very slow rate. I was happy that the awful, destructive ideas he had been expressing for so long were not a constant topic of conversation any more. Then suddenly, out of nowhere, I noticed Billy having very peculiar reactions to us and to his environment. We watched him closely and began to comprehend.

He seemed to be breaking through the darkness, the shadows that held him for so long. The walls were rolling away, and as the light of another existing world hit him, he was quite naturally blinded by it. He was in a state of shocked reality. It was all new and terrifying. He could not understand what was happening to him, and had no idea how to deal with it, as the phenomenon occurred again and yet again. He tried to balance himself emotionally, with one foot in each of his two worlds, not knowing whether to step forward to the new, or retreat to the safe old. At least that is the way it looked to us.

Billy had been ill all of his young life. He could not understand the alteration taking place within him as he was improving. During these days, he was more difficult to understand than usual, but we stuck with him. Normal people would not have encountered this, we knew, because they have what is called "a frame of reference." They know what it feels like to be well, as contrasted to not being so. In our child's case, he had no such frame of reference; therefore, the fluctuations taking place within his mind and body were very disturbing to him. The dismay and confusion he registered was perfectly understandable to us. In one sense it was the best bit of progress we could have hoped for, no matter how startling it looked to anyone else.

I reported our observations to his doctor on our next visit, and he said that many of his patients had similar problems as they improved. He told me it was a very trying time for them because of the stimulation to the brain resulting from the vitamin therapy. He mentioned that their hyperactivity increases during this time. I found this to be quite true with Billy. To help the boy, he prescribed a tranquilizer. When I protested, knowing what a regular tranquilizer did to Billy, he substituted another substance that had a quieting effect without the incessant movement that a regular tranquilizer always produced in our son. We found it to be a great help, and the boy calmed down and functioned much better.

During the summer of 1967, as we dealt with Billy's physical problems and adjusted his medication, we were still wrangling with the Board of Education about our son's scholastic future. We received several communications indicating their recommendations for school and treatment center placement. The first letter came from the advising psychiatrist of the Child Study Team. He suggested we look into a team learning center for emotionally sick, connected with a hospital not too far away. He was not aware that we had started Billy on the vitamin therapy nor of the progress he was making. Since my husband and I were both dead set against hospital treatment now, we didn't get excited about their letter, but my husband looked into it anyhow. He talked with the hospital administrators to find out what sort of program and treatment they offered. He was told that our son would be placed in a mixed ward of men and boys for several months. Then he would be completely analyzed and transferred to their teaching unit. Bill asked if they used vitamin therapy in the teaching unit or hospital, and was told no. That was all we had to hear.

In August we visited a Catholic school that was setting up a class for children with behavior disabilities. The class seemed well-run and better than almost any we had seen thus far. Unfortunately, they did not have state approval under the Beadleston Act as yet. This meant that Billy could not attend there and have his education paid for by the state. That school was out, but we kept on looking, for we were determined Billy should return to school the next fall.

Our third quest for a school for Billy was just as trying, just as frustrating, as the first two had been. The lack of facilities within our own state was discouraging. I told my aunt, who had taught for years in our local system, that I could not understand why nothing was available for children with problems like ours.

"It seems to me they have facilities for the retarded, the deaf, the blind—just about everything you can think of. Why don't they have more for kids like Billy? I am sure there are more like Billy; surely he is not *that* unique!" The system seemed woefully inadequate to me.

"Of course he isn't," she agreed, "and in a way he's less trouble than some other students I've had. I'll bet there are 'Billys' in every classroom in the system, but they are considered just problem kids, nothing more," she told me.

It didn't seem fair. I had to register a further protest while she listened.

"What burns me is that the only answer anyone seems to come up with is a residential or hospital setup. Sure, some need this, I admit; but not all. Why don't they have day schools especially for children with emotional problems? That way they are not torn away from their homes. They have to look to someone to give them security or stability somewhere along the line. I don't think sending them away is the complete answer. In Billy's case, I am *sure* of it." My aunt nodded in understanding.

"Yes, Jessie, but you must remember that some other families have more than one child to consider!"

I pondered that for a moment. What *if* Billy had had brothers and sisters? How could we have managed then?

"You know what I think?" I told her. "There should be several top-notch diagnostic centers throughout the state, where children who get into difficulties could be sent in their early years. If they were helped properly, early enough, then most of what we went through could have been avoided. And if a child is well enough to function in school, then there should be a school for him to go to. These special classes for emotionally disturbed are a stopgap, not a solution. Most of them are a hodgepodge of well-intentioned, but often poorly managed, programs. Look at what those two monstrous classes Billy was involved in did for him—absolutely nothing! More is needed, desperately needed, and I speak from experience." We weren't the only parents who cared—there must be thousands!

"What do you think you can do about it? You can't fight the whole school system for one child!" she said, in a tone of resignation.

"Ah, so many times I have felt like it, but maybe you're right." Maybe the school situation was hopeless. "At least he is improving, slowly, but improving. I guess I should be happy with that much, but I'm not. Children like my own left untreated or unhelped may become the eventual responsibility of the taxpayer. We have been fortunate in some ways. But wouldn't it make better sense, and be less expensive to solve the problem when the child is young? That way, many a burden could be lifted from the public's shoulders—and from the parents. Someday, with research, this problem will be eliminated entirely. Until then, why can't we provide more, sooner, when and where it is needed?" I was feeling like a real crusader.

But my aunt just shook her head and didn't answer me at all.

12

Calm Amid Storms

Billy advanced during August, 1967. He did not become perfectly normal overnight—far from it—but he did improve enough to want to return to school. Toward the end of the month, he asked us everyday if he could go back. He didn't want to stay home with a tutor any more. My husband got busy pounding on the door of the Board of Education without effect. Then he contacted the Commissioner of Education for the State of New Jersey, asking when the local board was going to do something about Billy's educational needs, since it was legally obligated to provide for our son's schooling.

Our first response from the local board was the one we expected. A tutor would be provided. We refused to accept this. Tutoring was inadequate, and Billy did not like the idea. Next we received a letter from the Assistant Director of Special Educational Services for the State of New Jersey. He said he was investigating the plans of our local board concerning our son's 1967-68 school year. We heard nothing further from anyone. Billy sat home with me as September passed. We were becoming annoyed at the delay. My husband had told the Assistant Director of the Board of Education about the vitamin therapy and how much better Billy was. We expected some immediate action.

One day Billy asked me why they didn't want him in school anymore, why he wasn't being treated like others. We were furious that our child was always suffering because of the lagging of decisions that had to made by those in authority.

Nevertheless, his father kept on hammering at doors until we were asked to have Billy's psychiatrist write his recommendations regarding the type of class he felt would help the child most. This request fulfilled, we sat and waited some more. Meanwhile, I taught Billy at home. Finally, after weeks of waiting, we wrote to our representative in the U.S. Congress, giving her the whole history of our son's case and questioning the present lack of cooperation we were facing. Ours was a simple request: put the child back in school; give him another chance!

October arrived, and my husband, who had been dealing with the Assistant Superintendent of Schools, was invited to appear before the local Child Study Team to explain Billy's medical program and his progress. Both of us went to the meeting. I did most of the talking, since my husband felt that I had found the treatment that was working for Billy.

For about forty minutes I described the substances Billy was taking, and the changes we had observed. I didn't claim he was perfect, just improved. The psychiatrist who was adviser to the Board took exception to some of my statements. He implied that the tranquilizers we were giving Billy would account for the changes we had observed in his behavior. When I asked him why I had noticed changes before the tranquilizer was introduced, he had no answer. The school psychologist mentioned again that all the harm had been done to our child in the first five years of his life.

My blood boiled, and I could not keep from expressing my rage. In a voice quavering with sarcasm, I said, "Will you please tell me what normal, concerned parents would deliberately raise or treat their only child in such a way as to purposely make him ill?" No answer was forthcoming. With that, the meeting broke up.

A short time later, a remedial learning specialist was sent to our home to observe Billy as he did his school work with me. Her first question was, "Does he always sit that still?"

Soon after, Billy had an interview with the psychiatrist who had been at the local Child Study Team meeting. Billy told the doctor he wanted to be back in class. The psychiatrist agreed to see what he could do about it, and commented to the boy that he was obviously overcoming a very great handicap.

I might add here that the two special teachers Billy had in the original special classes were no longer with the school system. I had heard that one was fired, and the other left to obtain more schooling. My judgment of them seemed to have been justified. They had been replaced by a man who was over six feet tall. It was in his group that Billy made his reentry into the local school system early in November.

The new teacher was well able to handle these children and maintain order in class. We weren't thrilled about Billy's placement, but since he had lost so much time, he could not very well be placed in a regular class now. Anything was better than having him remain at home with me any longer, especially since he now had the desire to return to his peers.

Billy had been out of a classroom for almost a year. The first few weeks he was apprehensive, thinking of his past experiences, but he was also pleased. This was perfectly natural and to be expected.

Recently I spoke to the man who was his teacher that

year. He told me the road back was difficult for my son, but there was steady progress. Billy was very hyperactive the first couple of months in class, but less so toward the middle of the school term. By the end of the year, his hyperactivity had ceased.

This year, the children were encouraged to express themselves freely in a constructive way. There was none of the damaging permissive behavior that had been allowed previously. Our son talked openly to his teacher about his feelings, problems, and the years he had suffered in those other classes. It was a new twist, a sorting out of his past frustrations. Talking helped him reorient his emotions. He recounted the fears and anxieties that had plagued him and talked to his teacher about us. He wanted to know why his parents had permitted him to suffer. At one point he told his teacher he wanted *him* for a father. He was very concerned that he might do us harm for failing him, that no one would stop him from behaving like Hitler, taking revenge on us all.

I have wondered many times if this attitude came about because we seldom punished Billy. We rarely spanked him, because if we did, he punished himself far more severely than necessary, sometimes verging on self-destruction. We wanted to avoid this tendency, so we usually talked to him, pointing out his transgression without attaching physical punishment to it.

One day in class during a discussion of this general nature, Billy became very angry with his teacher. He told the teacher he wanted to hit him. The teacher offered his arm to be struck, but Billy would not strike it. Then the teacher said to our son, "You see, Billy? You asked who would stop you from doing harm to others—and there's your answer. You stopped yourself. You answered your own question." Billy did not yet realize he could control his own impulses, but by this simple demonstration he began to see the truth.

Toward the end of this year, Billy once more became annoyed with the teacher, the class, the school. He told the instructor he was not coming to school anymore. In other words, he wanted to retreat temporarily. The teacher was wise, and knew a decision of this type should not be left to the child. He called me at home and told me to keep Billy with me a day or two; then he ordered my son to stay home the next day. I don't think Billy appreciated the fact that this decision was taken out of his hands. After spending the following day with me, he was more than willing to return to school. Billy made no further threats or complaints about attending class for the rest of the year.

This teacher did us another favor. He told me about a school that was extremely helpful and skilled at educating children like Billy. He suggested we look into it, as Billy was growing older and needed the companionship of children closer to his own age. I, too, felt my son was too old to continue where he was another year. He said that Billy was basically a student with a will to learn; but because he had been ill for years, it would take quite a while for him to catch up. He was not yet mature enough to accept the responsibility for his own success or failure. I agreed with his observations.

All around we were pleased with Billy's progress; and during February of this school year, we began to have further evidence that boosted our confidence in the megavitamin therapy.

Both Billy and his cousin are steam train buffs. Once a year, a group of people interested in transportation by this old-fashioned means run steam train excursions. Hordes of people go on these trips, and the tickets are usually sold out well in advance. Billy's cousin wanted to take him on this trip as a birthday gift. I wasn't keen on the idea of the two of them going alone—Billy might become upset—but we decided to take that chance. This particular journey was to take a route along the Jersey Central tracks to Wilkes-Barre, Pennsylvania, starting early on a Sunday morning and returning the same day.

I packed enough food for lunch and supper and put all Billy's pills in small bottles and put them in the food knapsack.

His father got up early and took him to the station, where he met his cousin, and there they waited. The train arrived late. That was the beginning of a long series of mishaps. They had the wrong type of coal to fire the engine, and all the way to Wilkes-Barre they had trouble. On the way back, the engine was derailed, and everyone was stuck in the middle of nowhere. The whole trip turned into a fiasco.

We did not know about any of this until my husband had made his fourth trip to the railroad station to meet the train. When no train arrived, he went to the police. Eventually the police informed the waiting parents and relatives that the train was stranded, our kids along with it.

I didn't sleep much, worrying about how Billy would take all this. In the end, all the people were returned home by bus, leaving the train in Pennsylvania. They had left our town about eight o'clock Sunday morning and didn't return until six o'clock the following morning.

Billy's cousin said Billy had behaved perfectly. He never let out a peep of complaint. They had been warm and had plenty to eat, thanks to Billy's well-stocked knapsack.

When Billy arrived home the next morning, he went

straight to bed and slept most of the day. After he awakened, he told me in detail all that had happened. He wasn't the least bit upset; in fact, he rather enjoyed the experience. It made me realize I could now trust him to accept the unusual, the unexpected, without falling apart—something I had never been able to do before.

The February train trip was an experience that showed his improvement, but in March he began upsetting us again. He would come home from school and fall on the sofa exhausted. He had put on a lot of weight during the months he had been at home with me, and I thought perhaps the extra weight was tiring him; but when I watched him closely, I changed my mind. The external inertia was accompanied by internal turmoil. He reminded me of a car with its motor running at full speed, out of gear, and standing still. Then, every once in a while, he would rush around, manifesting extreme distraction.

He was about due to visit his psychiatrist, so when the appointment date came, I told the doctor about my observations. First he said I should have Billy's blood tested. He ordered a six hour glucose tolerance test. Then, with the help of a metronome, he explained to Billy about the distortion of time sense or flow which frequently occurs in bio-chemical disorders. When the metronome was set at 180 beats per minute, Billy related that this was the speed at which ideas rushed through his head, and the speed he felt his body was going when he paced rapidly around. Billy himself set the metronome at 30 beats per minute and paced in slow motion, smiling as he said, "That's how it used to be, and I wish it would be that way again." He agreed that when his sense of time flow did slow down, he would no longer feel the need for outburst or pacing about.

We had the blood test done as soon as possible, and

to my heartbreaking sorrow, we learned that Billy too had diabetes mellitus. What else could go wrong for our child?

Our local doctor reexamined Billy and told me three things. First, he had to lose thirty pounds. Second, he had to be on a restricted diet. Of course I knew this from my own condition. The last thing was good news for a change. Billy would not have to take insulin, and his blood pressure had now dropped to a more normal level.

When our son was born, I knew there was a possibility of his developing diabetes, especially since his paternal grandfather and his aunt had the same illness. And so I had prepared him for this eventuality. Billy had often watched me taking my insulin, and I had talked to him about it. My husband did not like this idea. He felt there was no use burdening the child with more information on the subject than necessary. I did not agree, for if he was to become diabetic too, I wanted him to know what he would have to deal with.

Now my approach paid dividends. Billy was not upset or frightened when the doctor told him he was diabetic. The only question he asked was whether I would give him the shots if he had to take them. He accepted the restrictions of diet in the same way. Most children would have rebelled or cheated—not Billy.

Once in a while, when I look at him now and think of all he has been through and accepted as his lot, I know what a truly fine person he is. How strong is his will to survive! I often wonder how many adults could have endured all he endured and come out with hope in their hearts.

We succeeded in getting his weight down during the rest of the school year and the following summer. We looked forward to that summer for two reasons. First,

Billy was better, and secondly, we had bought a new and bigger boat. Now that we all had our sea legs, and were beginning to relax a bit, we felt we all deserved a little pleasure out of life.

My husband had purchased a twenty-six-foot fiber glass cabin cruiser which Billy christened *The Falcon*. We were going to hunt the bay, he said, and he was going to be chief pirate. We ate, slept, and lived on the boat every weekend and during our vacation. While at the shore, Billy did fairly well. He did not get close to any of the other children, but the people were all nice and understanding toward him. He was accepted, with no questions asked.

One afternoon we had all been swimming in a favorite spot halfway down the bay. This place had a sandy beach, and boats could be brought in close to shore. The afternoon passed quickly, but the sky suddenly began to darken and look threatening. Since our boat could only be driven from the flying bridge, we decided to head back to the dock before the approaching storm broke. We raced up the bay, and just as we passed inside the breakwater, the storm came crashing down directly overhead. The rain, driven by a fifty mile per hour wind, fell with such force that we could not see three feet in front of the bow. There we were, in our bathing suits, pelted by hailstones and ice cold rain. I shooed Billy into the cabin and grabbed my raincoat and my husband's. As we approached our slip, my husband yelled down for me to grab the lines we had strung on either side of our docking space with the metal boat hook, but I couldn't. The rain and hail were beating into my face with such force that I couldn't see, let alone get hold of any lines, no matter how hard I tried.

The lightning crackled wildly over our heads, and the thunder reverberated with a deafening roar. Beneath my raincoat I was shaking with cold and fright. I don't know how my husband stayed on that unprotected bridge. Each time the lightning flashed, I was sure he'd be hit, for we had to keep circling inside the breakwater, and there was no place to tie up. The wind kept gusting with such force we could not back the boat into the slip. Every time we came around, it blew us in the opposite direction. Even with full throttle we made no headway. It seemed to me that hours passed. The storm was so savage, I thought we would all be struck dead any second.

As we made another pass near our dock, we were about ten feet, perhaps less, from a sailboat. Just as we were turning away from the sailboat, there was a blinding flash of light followed by thunder so loud I stumbled on the boat deck. At the same time that the light flashed, I heard my husband give out a terrific cry. I thought he was struck, but I looked up to the bridge and he was still clinging there. As cold and wet as I was, I began to sweat, and I don't mean to perspire! Finally there was a lull—just long enough for us to dock the boat with both of us working full speed. Then the second wave of the storm hit.

When my husband came down from the bridge, his eyes were red as fire. I thought they were bleeding, but they weren't—just bloodshot. He told me he received a terrible shock from the controls during that one awful crash. I just said a small prayer of thanksgiving that the ordeal was over.

We had been lucky—and then some—but we did not realize it until the next day when we learned that the worst stroke of lightning had struck the sailboat as we were passing. It had stripped the mast top, wrecked the mast guy wires, and burned fire spots on the ship's hull. We learned, too, that all the people in their docked boats had been watching us struggling until the rain came down so hard they could no longer see us. All the while, we were circling between ten and fifteen feet away from them. After our boat was secured, I had felt heavy, and looked down at my vinyl raincoat. Both of my pockets were sticking out as though stuffed with air-filled balloons. They were overflowing with ice and water! That was quite a storm!

What was Billy doing all this time? He was inside the cabin, nonchalantly reading a comic book, without a fear or care in the world. When I thought about how he acted on our plane trip to California, and how unimpressed he was by the outrage of the storm we had just survived, I couldn't believe he was the same boy.

Other than the storm, we experienced only one bad time throughout the whole summer of 1968. For several days Billy had complained of not feeling just right. He did not complain of being sick at his stomach; instead, he said he had the jitters. We watched him become more and more agitated over things he had not discussed with us for months. It was as though a culmination of horror was suddenly hitting him, and all of the past years' skeletons came rattling out of his emotional closet for a disturbing *danse macabre*.

He talked in review for three days, and kept asking what was happening to him. In some ways his behavior corresponded to that which had preceded his first siege of vitamin poisoning. He raved on, catapulting from old thoughts to new ones. He couldn't keep up with his changing mental patterns. There was no time for mental adjustment.

I had noticed that after Billy had lost weight on his diabetic diet his medications appeared to be working more effectively. This was undoubtedly contributing to the rapid and violent personality change we saw in him then. It was unlike any we had observed in him before.

We called his psychiatrist and explained what was wrong. He told me Billy was changing too rapidly, and needed to be slowed down. His body was pushing him in a direction he was not yet emotionally prepared for. Following his advice, we stopped all medication for a short time, and Billy recovered. He rapidly pulled out of this temporary upset. Then we started to reintroduce certain substances gradually again. It did the trick.

13

The Happy Time

During the winter of 1968, while Billy was attending the new special class in the public school system, we investigated the day school his teacher had recommended. Although the class he was attending was a great improvement over the first two, it was still inadequate, and the pupils were younger than he was. Fourteen years old, Billy didn't like the idea of spending another year with "babies."

Lord Stirling School, a private institution, accepts only students referred to them by the public school system. A student must have at least average intelligence and must be able to relate to some type of educational program. Enrollment consists of twenty-seven boys and five girls, representing 17 school districts. The schoolhouse is a rather tired old farm building, but the physical facilities seem unimportant compared to what goes on inside the school.

The place has an atmosphere the kids love. Mr. John Aylward, the director, is a young, progressive-thinking psychologist who knows what he is doing. His school is one of the very few in New Jersey that accepts emotionally maladjusted students over twelve on a day school basis. He calls his establishment a psycho-educational center for children with behavioral disabilities. He and his teachers work with the students, using a very personal, involved, relationship therapy. They accept the students for what they are, as they are, working to bring about behavior modification, educating the student at the same time. Medication and formal therapy are left to the parents of the child. By carefully screening the students before they are accepted, they are able to do the most good possible for each individual.

They make each child feel like a worthwhile human being. Many come to the school having been rejected by society. They feel that not much is expected of them in the way of acceptable behavior, because they believe they are worthless. When the child begins to know he is more than nothing, he starts to respond.

The pupils learn that people care about them and their individuality. The teacher's personal involvement with the students encourages them to share and expose their innermost feelings, good and bad. As the years of submerged repressions bubble to the surface, changes for the better begin to take place.

Thanks to the vitamin therapy, our son was now well enough to respond to this type of atmosphere. We decided to ask the Board of Education to make application for Billy's enrollment in Lord Stirling School.

They moved swiftly this time, and Billy's application was accepted for the following year. Since their enrollment was restricted to thirty-two students, we were anxious to attend to the matter as early as possible. The way Billy handled his personal interview with Mr. Aylward was rewarding to me. It was entirely different from our disastrous experience in the out-of-state treatment center. I had often thought of how Providence took over then. Their refusal to take our son was a blessing in disguise.

When Billy started to attend Lord Stirling School he

was both timid and apprehensive. He took his old hang-ups and some of his fears along with him, but slowly we watched the old feelings and attitudes break down and change. If someone bothered him, he still went to his teacher for protection. After several months, he dealt with the other child directly, without the aid of a mediator. He actually defended himself!

Billy's hypochondriac symptoms vanished. On occasion I even had to remind him to attend to certain essentials, as mothers of normal boys have to now and then. Whenever I got after him he called me a nag! How perfectly normal! At the same time, he began to accept constructive criticism without an accompanying emotional explosion. He began to show signs of taking the pressures of everyday living with relative ease.

A new attitude began to bud in his schoolwork too. He no longer begged us for help, but stated that he was capable of doing things himself. We agreed. At this point we were not overly concerned with his scholastic progress. There is no value in possessing a storehouse of knowledge and facts if you cannot communicate or relate to others. Our greatest delight was in seeing Billy begin to respond and interact with others. He was gradually getting the idea that feeling for others is as important as interest in ourselves. Although Billy's manners did not necessarily reflect his changing personality, we tried not to criticize him for every breach of etiquette. We were more eager to build his confidence.

Billy stopped complaining about noise, and loudness no longer sent him into a tailspin. He turned the stereo on full blast without batting an eye. He became less hesitant about trying something new. Change no longer offered a threat, but was approached with interest. Oh, he daydreamed in class sometimes, but he no longer lived in a world of fantasy, darkness and despair. Most important of all, he no longer talked incessantly about the terrible suffering he endured at the hands of the boy who drove him wild. To me this meant he was not constantly thinking about his unhappy past. He could forgive! And the ability to forgive himself and others was surely required for his wholeness.

One afternoon he came home from school very proud of himself and handed me two stories he had written. "Here, Mom, read these," he said.

"All right, Billy," I said, taking the papers and sitting down to read them. "Did you write these yourself?"

"Yes, I did," he said, "and I want to make sure you read them."

The first theme was about a boy who had schizophrenia. He was so ill that he did not understand what his own image should be; he had no mental picture of himself. The second theme described the tormented thoughts of someone who felt like Hitler, wanting to destroy everyone and everything in the world. The story concluded with the admission that the boy was relating what had gone on inside his head when he was very ill. Today, it said, that boy no longer felt that way. It was plain to me that Billy was writing about himself.

"Billy, your stories are excellent," I told him. "Tell me, is that the way you used to feel inside, when you got so upset sometimes?"

His eyes were shining, and he nodded his head vigorously.

"Yes, Mom, but that's all over and past, and I never want to be like that again!"

My own eyes were swimming with tears—of joy.

"Don't worry, Billy, it won't ever come back! I know!"

After that day almost all of his stories showed a new and different twist. He stopped talking about Hitler or comparing himself to him. Now he makes jokes about the man. He even gave away all his pictures of German war leaders, equipment, and everything else pertaining to the German army during World War II. If he reads or talks about that part of history it is strictly from a historical point of view! Quite a change! He has switched to writing about Charlie Chaplin or some other screen character, with humor and happy endings thrown in. All this reflects his new control over his daydream world and his changing concept of himself. Even his drawings indicate his tremendous sense of humor.

While this marvelous revolution was taking place, we continued to take Billy for his monthly visits to his psychiatrist, increasing or adjusting Billy's medication according to his instructions. By the end of May, 1968, our son was taking eleven different substances. His psychiatrist had substituted a new one to take the place of niacinamide, which was taken in such large quantities it sometimes upset Billy's stomach. The new substance provided the same benefits, but did not produce any undesirable side effects. At that time it was not on the open market, but we used it for a year or more and it worked well for Billy. Unfortunately, for some reason I do not understand, his psychiatrist can no longer obtain it, and we now have to go to Canada for the same thing.

At any rate, our son was so greatly improved that his doctor gradually lowered the dosages, and even eliminated some of Billy's medication until he took only two pills a day. As events continued to go well, I had to pinch myself to realize this was our son. He was a pleasure to have about the house, and very helpful. He did many chores willingly, volunteering to wash or dry the supper dishes. His whole attitude toward almost everything was a testimonial to the good I knew was always within him.

One evening in the winter Billy sat down to watch a television movie, "Bird Man of Alcatraz." Usually he was only superficially interested in motion pictures, but this night he sat quietly, completely absorbed in what was taking place on the set. I was busy elsewhere; so was his father. When the movie was over, he came to talk to us about it. He was impressed, not with the fact that a man had spent most of his life in solitary confinement for murder, but with what the man had done with this time. He had learned several languages. He had studied the illnesses and habits of birds and taught himself how to take care of them. He made a tremendous contribution to the scientific field with his research while he was imprisoned. Our son was elated with the way in which this person had overcome his fate.

"You know, Mom, Pop, I was just thinking," he said. "If *he* can do it, so can I. He wasn't useless after all." Billy sounded so encouraged and happy.

His father replied, "We know you can do it, Billy. We have every faith and trust in you. Everything *will* be fine, and you are going to have a wonderful and productive life." This wasn't just lip service or wishful thinking now. We *did* know.

I was impressed, too, with my son's new determination. We always knew he "had it in him," but now he was starting to express his positive thoughts. The pendulum of his life was swinging in the right direction at last. His social life was taking a turn for the better too, with a new activity. Every Saturday afternoon during the winter of 1968-69, he went bowling with a group of exceptional children. Some of these youngsters were retarded, and some had physical disabilities, but to watch them was a feast for the eyes. They did better than some "normal" bowlers I have watched. Billy enjoyed himself and looked forward to his Saturday afternoons out.

Our upward climb continued until February of 1969. It was like living in paradise, but sometimes paradise has a dormant volcano that suddenly erupts. Our volcano was rumbling, but we were so pleased with Billy's progress that we did not foresee its immediate eruption! Towards the end of the month, I noticed Billy was becoming edgy again; some subtle symptoms were returning. I mentioned my feeling to my husband, but before we could discuss it thoroughly, Billy came home from school one day and started behaving strangely.

"Will they send me back to the public schools, Mom?" he asked me.

"What do you mean, Billy?" An alarm rang inside of me—I knew something was terribly wrong. "What's the matter? What makes you ask me that? Did something happen in school today?"

"Yes," he answered, "something happened in school all right, and I am not satisfied with myself at all." He hung his head.

"Can you tell me about it?" I asked, trying to keep my voice from reflecting my panic.

"I can't," he said. "I'm too ashamed." He wouldn't let his eyes look at me, just stared at the floor.

With that, I headed for the telephone to call his teacher. As I approached the phone, it started to ring. It was his teacher calling me.

"Mrs. Foy, I called because I have noticed a letdown, a backsliding, in Billy's condition. Today was the worst day we have had with him since he entered the school." I could tell his teacher was deeply concerned.

"Yes, I know," I stammered. "I was just on my way to call you. Billy came home very upset—but he can't tell me what happened." I paused.

"Well, in class this morning," the teacher began, "Billy put his lunch on the desk, and the bag fell over. His thermos bottle broke, spilling milk all over the place. Billy picked up the bag and hurled it into the waste-basket, kicking and screaming and crying the whole time. No one could do a thing with him the rest of the day." There was a silence while the full significance of Billy's behavior penetrated my mind.

"It's too bad we didn't talk sooner," I said. "I've noticed myself that Billy's condition has been deteriorating the past two weeks. I'll call his psychiatrist to see if his medication needs to be increased." That seemed to me to be the first action to take. *Oh, we couldn't begin having trouble again!*

The teacher had something else to tell me.

"Did you know, too, that he has been throwing away his pills lately?" she asked. "He tells me he thinks they're giving him side effects, as they did once before."

My heart sank.

"No, I didn't know about the pills," I said. "Thank you for letting me know." I wondered why I hadn't been notified sooner. Perhaps we could have forestalled this relapse.

There was still more to be told. "He hasn't eaten his lunch for the past two days either," the teacher said.

I didn't think the lack of food would hurt him, but the rest had to be attended to immediately.

When she hung up, I called Billy's psychiatrist, who increased the dosage to thirteen pills a day, beginning immediately. Within twenty-four hours, Billy returned to acceptable normal behavior. To our minds this was absolute proof that his problem had a bio-chemical basis.

After the crisis had passed, I talked with Billy about it.

"How do you feel now, Billy?" I began.

"Oh, much better—just fine!" He seemed surprised that I had asked.

"Billy, I cannot overemphasize the importance of taking those pills. They mean the difference between life and death for you. If you don't feel right, come and tell me or your Dad, but don't let matters get so far out of hand again." I repressed an involuntary shudder.

"But, Mom, I thought they were giving me side effects again, and I couldn't take that!" Even in the midst of my concern I could be thankful that Billy was defending himself.

"Look, sweetheart," I told him, "you are not the doctor, so why don't you leave those decisions up to him? Don't try to doctor yourself—just come to us if you are puzzled or feel peculiar. That's what we are here for—to help you." I could tell that he understood, and that he was sorry for any distress he had caused us.

"Okay, okay. It won't happen again," he promised.

He had been doing so well for so long that we had started to take things for granted, a costly mistake we would never repeat.

His teacher wrote me a note the day after his vitamin intake had been increased. She was amazed at the spontaneous improvement that had taken place in him during that one night. She had really been alarmed the day he misbehaved, for she had never seen him like that before. Later, at a P.T.A. meeting, I told her that this sort of thing used to occur ten or twenty times a day when he was very ill. She just looked at me stunned, marveling that we had survived it. Sometimes I marveled too.

Billy himself was overjoyed by his improvement. After this upset, he continued to improve. The director of his school told me several times that it was rewarding to see the strides Billy was making. He couldn't have been more pleased with him. When our son had first begun to attend Lord Stirling School, he was awkward at almost everything. He couldn't even run properly. He was poor at playing games with other boys, and didn't know how to socialize with them. Slowly, but surely, he was advancing in every area of development.

His class planned a trip to Stokes State Forest at the end of the school year 1969. This was the first time Billy was to be away from us since his ill-fated trip to Expo 1967. I was anxious, as usual, for the class was going to be away three days and two nights. I could have saved myself the trouble of worrying; Billy had the time of his life. He slept in a room with two other boys, and in the daytime they roamed the forest together. Mr. Aylward said it was sheer joy to watch Billy laughing and playing with friends.

At one time on the trip, his teacher told me, Billy was talking to another boy about an imaginary character he had created. The other boy told him that what he was saying was "nuts." Billy looked at his critic and retorted, "You're wrong! That's not 'nuts'! I just happen to have a very creative imagination!" With that they both laughed. And the other boy looked at my son with new respect and admiration.

The first thing Billy said when he came home was, "Boy, I wish I had a brother or sister. I'm going to miss the other kids. Who wants to be all alone anyhow? It's just too lonesome being an only child." I rejoiced, remembering all the years when other people had not mattered to him at all.

"I'm sorry, Billy," I said, "but you do have five cousins, and they'll have to be your brothers. Anyhow, school is nearly over for this year, and we'll be going down to the shore soon. You'll have plenty of company

there." We were all looking forward to a joyful holiday
this year.

Near the last day of school, Billy went into the
bathroom to weigh himself. From the bathroom he proceeded to the kitchen, where he looked into the cabinet
containing his pills. From there he went to his room.
For a few moments I tried to figure out what he was
doing. My built-in alarm system began to jangle.

"What are you doing, Billy?" I called out. "Is something wrong? What's bothering you?" My skin began to
feel clammy. But Billy just laughed at me.

"Oh, Mom," he chided. "I was just wondering why I
am feeling so well these days."

With that I laughed out loud too, and said a silent
prayer of thanks. I had waited fifteen years to hear my
child say that to me.

From that day to this, Billy has been saying and
doing things that bring warmth to our days and gladness
to our hearts.

We spent most of our vacation at the shore on our
boat. The summer was all we had hoped it would be.
Billy began to blossom into a social butterfly. He talked
to everyone about everything, and hopped from boat to
boat, visiting friends, and enjoying life to the fullest.

One night we were in charge of club activities. It was
card night. Billy helped me with the refreshments and
played checkers with another boy without any self-con-
sciousness, and with obvious enjoyment.

Another night we all went to visit one of the
members of our group who had rented a cottage for two
weeks. Billy played with all the children and later said
to me, "Gee, Mom, those kids really *like* me!" This fact
seemed to surprise him.

"Of *course* they do, Billy," I said. "You're a nice boy
to know!" He was tickled pink! We were delighted too.

He was growing in spirit and confidence and learning, all at the same time.

When we are at the coast, Billy spends a great deal of time with his father. He looks up to him for guidance, instruction, and for the image of what a man should be. I leave them alone, for I know Billy should follow the example set by his father. Who wants to hang on his mother's apron strings anyhow? Certainly not a fifteen-year-old boy! Billy and his Dad talk, ride bikes, swim, and work on and handle the boat together. I enjoy the air, the water, and the people—but my greatest pleasure lies in watching my son become well. Once in a while, however, I stick my nose in and do something with Billy alone.

It was toward the end of the season when Billy and I decided to take a walk together without his dad. Near the boat yard is a large bridge, which connects our side of the bay with a strip of land that divides the bay from the ocean. We enjoy walking over the bridge, and then along the ocean shore, especially when there are not too many people about. We started out early in the evening. The bright summer sun was fading, but the air was soft and warm. At this hour the traffic that hums over the bridge all day had slowed down, and it was relatively quiet, except for the sound of the moving water.

To cross the bridge, we had to proceed along a narrow sidewalk, not wide enough for two people to walk side by side. We strolled along, one behind the other, Indian fashion. We were approaching the arch of the bridge, enjoying the view of the sky, the water, and the boats passing underneath us, when I felt my son touching my shoulder. I thought he was going to call my attention to a large yacht that was heading up the waterway toward us, but he fooled me. Instead, he came close to my side and put his arm around me. Almost silently, he whispered to me, "Thanks, Mom, thanks for everything!" I knew what he meant, and I was deeply touched. Those simple words had more meaning for me than the greatest oratory in the world. It was the most gratifying moment of my whole life to know that he appreciated our support all those years.

From then on we laughed, talked, and played while we were heading for the beach. We took off our shoes and made patterns in the sand, happier than we had ever been before—happy in our newly found peace, happy in being together, happy in Billy's good health.

We lingered a long time along the water's edge, watching the setting sun glow red in the sky and seeing its reflected brilliance dance upon the water. Then we headed back to the boat yard. I was deep in thought, reviewing all we had been through and wondering what the future held.

Mentally, I recorded a chronology of the improvements Billy was displaying. The way he talked and expressed his ideas was first on a long list. Billy, a friend, and I were walking down one of the docks one night, and the moon was shining as bright as daylight. Billy looked up and said, "Well, Mom, there is the sun of the night!"

The friend turned to Billy and said, "Billy, you have poetry in you. You must get it from your mother." I laughed. I don't consider myself a poet.

"He's got a lot of his father in him too, you know!" I countered. Then Billy laughed.

Our son was becoming a smooth composite of thought and action, not a disjointed, shattered personality. He is taking in all his experiences with his eyes, his ears—all his senses—and relating one to another, integrating information. He is learning how to relate one step to another. He is learning how to study, absorb, and use his knowledge in all areas of living. He is expressing emotion with greater ease, without rancor, fear, and confusion. He is learning to care about his fellowman and learning how to get along with him.

Some of these qualities were evidenced the July night the Apollo 11 landed on the moon. Billy watched the whole event on television, from blast-off to splashdown. The night the astronauts walked on the moon, he stayed up until they were safely back in the Eagle. He wanted to make sure nothing went wrong.

While I was reviewing all this, I turned my thoughts to what was ahead. The next step was the beginning of the 1969 school year.

Before starting school this year, Billy had spoken to his father about his mixed-up education. He was worrying about the years he had lost, and wondered if he would ever be able to make them up.

"Do you think what I have learned so far is good enough, Pop?" He didn't sound discouraged, merely curious about it.

"Of course, Billy. What you have learned so far is fine." His father radiated confidence at him. "Don't forget, education is more than what we read in books; it's living too. Besides, you are young yet, and have plenty of time ahead to learn everything you should know. Education has nothing to do with calendar age, Billy. Some people go to school much later in life. There's no time limit set on learning."

Billy nodded his head.

"If you say so, I believe you. And don't worry, Pop, I'll keep trying. I know everything is going to be okay now; nothing is wrong. Because I am well now, not sick any more."

With that attitude in mind, he entered school in the fall.

The other night we went to the first P.T.A. meeting of the year and heard the best report on our son we have had the pleasure of listening to since he was born. He is doing well, and his teachers are thrilled with him, just as we are. He is taking the initiative and accepting responsibility for his action, and for his success or failure. His teacher told me he sat down and wrote a story in German for her, without being asked to do so. She was surprised. She also told us he is getting along well with the other children. He is a bit sensitive once in a great while, but his general responsiveness to his peers is really rewarding. He is comfortable and at ease with them.

While we were at the school that evening, Mr. Aylward told me about a humorous conversation he had with Billy. Once a week he has a "small talk" session with our son. During the same afternoon, the rest of the boys are taking a course in sex education, taught by another man teacher. When Billy went to see Mr. Aylward this particular day, he said, "Do you think we could hurry our talk up today, Mr. Aylward? I don't want to be late for sex this afternoon."

Mr. Aylward was puzzled for an instant, and then broke into laughter. "Billy," he chuckled, "I think what you mean is you don't want to be late for the sex education class. Is that right?"

"Sure, that's what I mean," Billy replied.

"Sometimes, Mrs. Foy, that boy of yours can be very funny!"

14

The Last Hurrah!

We have finally chased the darkness from Shadows' child. He is released from their imprisoning power. He now belongs to this world, and to us, his parents. He is our son. We are living in the light of God's world with him at last.

I do not think anyone can comprehend what this means unless they have lived as we did for fourteen years. This past summer was the happiest, most rewarding, most fulfilling experience imaginable for all of us. During the first two years Billy was on the vitamin therapy, I used to say to his psychiatrist that I could see improvement, but I was not completely satisfied. I knew he was better, but, to me, there was a last step to be conquered. He had not overcome the small traces of darkness remaining, or reached the complete clarity of pure light I hoped would come. I know now we have reached this stage, and that he will make it all the way. Of course there are no guarantees in life, or in medicine, but I do know that this simple treatment brought a very ill child from the brink of oblivion back to functioning as a human being.

Some will argue that Billy may have recovered spontaneously, as sometimes happens with schizophrenics. Some will say he might have improved through a natu-

ral maturing as he grew older, but he had already started to change physically when he was at his lowest ebb.

We had tried all the conventional psychological
methods of treatment, with fruitless results, before using
the vitamins. I believe that without them, we would
have lost our son forever. I say this unequivocally;
nothing could convince me otherwise.

How do I feel about this megavitamin treatment for
schizophrenics? How does one feel about a gift from
God?

Gone is Shadows' child!

We welcome the morning—when all things are made
new.

Epilogue

Perhaps when you have read this story, you will wonder why a mother would have wanted to tell it. My reasons for writing this book were simple ones. I felt very deeply that there must be other mothers and fathers struggling with similar problems throughout this world, and they should be told of our experiences so that they could avoid the pitfalls into which we fell. I certainly wish I had had such a book when my child was growing up.

Another reason was simply gratitude to both man and God. I wanted the chance to give back to others part of what we have received in living with this problem. God sustained me in many ways, and I found relief from my burdens through prayer—oh, not formal church prayer always, but just talking to Him as I worked and went about the business of daily living. My son was always on my mind, and what hurt him, hurt us. I found by praying quietly, sometimes just saying a thank you when a day went right, that I felt happier and less distressed than I thought possible.

I found that work helped me too. My little job got me away long enough to let me relax and think about something else. I came home from my labors refreshed, and ready to tackle what came next.

In the final analysis, my thanks must also go to the men who, through their research and faith, found that there was help for children afflicted as ours was.

Recently I allowed Billy to read this manuscript.

"What do you think about it, Billy?" I asked him. "Have I told our story the way it happened?"

"Yes, Mother," he answered. "But when I read it, it was like reading about someone else—not me as I feel today."

Although he accepted the book as his story, Billy seemed troubled in the next day or so—troubled, not in the old way, not with any recurrence of symptoms of his sickness, but as if he was evaluating himself. He hadn't liked looking at the picture of what he had been. It was too ugly. It *wasn't* the way he felt now—but it *was* the way he *had* been. He seemed puzzled, as if wondering what to do about it. I had nothing to offer him . . .

But Billy wasn't blind. He had seen that I had received great sustenance from my belief in God.

And suddenly, one afternoon, Billy asked his father to take him to church. No, he didn't want to wait until Sunday; he wanted to go right then.

His father raised his eyebrows and looked quizzically at me. I nodded, wondering just what Billy had in mind.

They drove to the church and Billy went inside by himself. He remained there alone for nearly half an hour. When he came out, the troubled look was gone. It had been replaced by a look of peace and joy.

"What did you do in there, Billy?" his father asked him.

"I just prayed, is all," Billy answered. "And it's all right now. The bad times are *gone*—not just *past,* but *gone.*" There was a beautiful finality to what he said.

Later, when my husband told me what had happened, I realized that Billy must have accepted God's forgiveness for himself, accepted it so fully and unconditionally it was as if the bad times had never been!

The next Sunday he accompanied his father to church—for the first time in years. We knew it took great courage for him to go back, but he was equal to it. He sang the hymns and prayed the prayers with the rest of the congregation. And when the service was over and they were leaving the sanctuary, Billy spoke cordially to everyone who spoke to him. His face shone with happiness and wholeness!

As I write this now, in the week following that Sunday, I can see the wholeness, the newness, still shining in him. It's as if "Shadows' child" has been *completely* taken away, and in his place is the person God intended for Billy to be from the very beginning.

Our whole family rejoices now, secure in the truth it took us so long to learn. Billy had had an insight into it years ago when he thought that the act of confirmation would accomplish his healing:

"I am the Lord that healeth thee." (Exodus 15:26)

A little child has led us, and I thank the Lord that He has answered our every prayer, above all we could ask or think.

If this very personal and often painful revelation helps only one other victim of this horrendous illness to find his way back to health, then it has been worth every moment we have struggled through, every heartbreaking, tragic moment we relived to write it.

We are so proud of our beloved son, whose unselfishness and bravery have made this book possible.

> But if we hope for that we see not,
> then do we with patience wait for it.
> *Romans 8:25*

References

Beers, Clifford. *A Mind That Found Itself*. Doubleday, 1908.

Landis, Carney. *Varieties of Psychopathological Experience*. Holt, Rinehart & Winston, 1964.

Lorenz, Sarah E. *And Always Tomorrow*. Holt, Rinehart & Winston, 1963.

Schreber, Daniel. *Memoirs of My Nervous Illness*. London: William Dawson & Sons, Ltd., 1955.

Sommer, Robert, and Osmond, Humphry. "Autobiographies of Former Mental Patients." Reprinted from *Journal of Mental Science*, CVI, No. 443 (April 1960).

Wilson, L. *This Stranger My Son*. Putnam, 1967.